THE HIKERS COMPANION FOR BEGINNERS

ESSENTIAL TIPS AND TRICKS FOR HIKING WITH CONFIDENCE

QUINN MARSHAL

TABLE OF CONTENTS

MEDICAL DISCLAIMER

The information provided in this book is for educational and informational purposes only. It is not intended to replace professional medical advice, diagnosis, or treatment. Always consult with a qualified healthcare provider before making any changes to your hiking or outdoor activities, especially if you have pre-existing medical conditions or are taking medications.

The author and publisher of this book are not healthcare professionals and do not provide medical advice. The content presented in this book is based on research, personal experiences, and general knowledge about hiking and outdoor activities. However, each individual's health and circumstances are unique, and what works for one person may not work for another.

The activities, techniques, and suggestions described in this book carry inherent risks. Hiking and outdoor activities can be physically demanding and may pose potential dangers and hazards. It is essential to assess your own physical capabilities, fitness level, and health status before engaging in any activities discussed in this book.

The author and publisher of this book disclaim any liability, loss, or risk incurred as a direct or indirect consequence of using the information presented in this book. They shall not be held responsible for any injuries, accidents, or damages that may occur during hiking or outdoor activities.

Please consult with a qualified healthcare professional, such as a physician or a certified wilderness medicine expert, for personalized medical advice regarding your specific health condition, fitness level, and suitability for engaging in hiking or outdoor activities. They are the best resource to provide guidance based on your individual needs and circumstances.

By reading this book and engaging in any activities described within, you acknowledge and accept the inherent risks associated with hiking and outdoor activities. You assume full responsibility for your actions, and the author and publisher shall not be held liable for any consequences arising from your participation in such activities.

Remember, safety should always be the top priority during any outdoor adventure. Use common sense, follow safety guidelines, and seek professional advice when necessary.

INTRODUCTION

There is an innate allure that beckons us to explore the great outdoors, immerse ourselves in the beauty of nature, and embark on journeys that challenge and inspire. Hiking—the timeless art of traversing landscapes on foot—has captivated human beings for centuries. From rugged mountain peaks to serene forest trails, hiking offers a pathway to discovery, self-reflection, and a profound connection with the natural world.

The Hiker's Companion is an invitation to embrace the wanderer within, step outside the boundaries of everyday life, and embark on an unforgettable adventure along the trails less traveled. In this book, we'll delve into the heart of hiking, uncovering the myriad reasons why people of all ages, genders, and backgrounds find solace, joy, and plain old fun in the act of putting one foot in front of the other.

Hiking is quickly becoming one of the most popular outdoor activities, due in part to the awareness that social media platforms create, with approximately 57.8 million hikers in the US alone. While everyone's reasons for hiking may differ, we all come together under the same sky to marvel at the beauty of nature. With no minimum or maximum distance one must travel to hike, your only limit is how far your feet can carry you. A successful hike is not measured by how far or how high you can go but by the quality of the experience and its impact on your life.

Hiking has an attraction that resonates with adventurers and nature enthusiasts alike. One of the greatest joys of hiking is the sheer freedom it offers. On the trail, our minds are liberated; we escape the clutches of our screens and the daily grind, slowing the relentless pace of modern life to find solace and serenity amidst the grandeur of mountains, valleys, and meandering streams. Each step taken is an opportunity to leave the hustle and bustle behind and embrace the simplicity and purity of the natural world.

Beyond freedom, hiking grants us a sense of accomplishment and empowerment. Each hill climbed, each summit conquered, and each rugged trail overcome strengthens not only our physical endurance but also our mental resilience. The challenges encountered on the trail often mirror the obstacles we face in life, and through hiking, we learn to confront them with determination, perseverance, and grace.

Hiking is a journey of self-discovery and introspection. As we navigate through varied landscapes, we have time to reflect on our thoughts, dreams, and aspirations. The rhythmic motion of walking opens the door to deeper contemplation and creativity, allowing us to connect with our innermost selves and find clarity amidst the chaos.

The lure of hiking is also fueled by the promise of discovery and exploration. Every trail is a gateway to new vistas, hidden waterfalls, ancient ruins, and abundant wildlife. With every bend and turn, a sense of wonder unfolds, and we find ourselves lost in the enchanting stories whispered by the winds and the murmurs of the earth.

Hiking provides us with an opportunity to foster bonds and build meaningful connections with fellow trekkers. When sharing the trail with kindred spirits, we unite under a common love for nature, camaraderie, and shared experiences. The friendships formed on the trail often transcend boundaries, reminding us of the universal spirit that connects all humanity.

In this guide, we will embark on a holistic exploration of hiking, encompassing the essence of various hiking types, from day hikes to challenging multiday backpacking adventures. We will delve into the ancient knowledge of navigating by map and compass, how to stay healthy and safe, how to deal with wildlife and the elements, hiking etiquette, and much more, ensuring that you can savor the thrill of hiking responsibly and sustainably.

During the course of this guide, I hope to ignite the spark of adventure within your soul and entice you to don your hiking boots and embark on an extraordinary journey of self-discovery and connection with the natural world. The trails await, and the possibilities are endless; take the first step and dive into the realm of hiking—a realm where wanderlust is awakened, and every path is a new adventure!

1

HIKING 101

I took a walk in the woods and came out taller than the trees.

— HENRY DAVID THOREAU

WHAT IS HIKING?

Hiking is a recreational activity that involves walking or trekking on trails or paths, usually in natural environments such as forests, mountains, parks, or countryside areas. It allows the exploration, discovery, and appreciation of the beauty of nature.

Hiking is an escape into the wilderness that fosters a deeper connection to the natural world and a greater appreciation for the comforts you leave behind. As you journey away from civilization with nothing but the gear on your back, it's also a journey of self-discovery that can be physically and mentally challenging at times.

DIFFERENT TYPES OF HIKING

There is a type of hiking to suit just about everyone's needs or skill level with few rules that are set in stone. Let's have a look at some of them, starting with the three most popular types of hiking.

Day Hiking

Day hiking involves shorter hikes that are 8–10 miles long and typically last 3–10 hours. The length of time the hike takes can vary depending on the season and location, but a day hiker has no intention of spending the night outdoors. Very little gear is needed on a day hike besides footwear and water.

The starting point of a typical day hike is a designated trail-head or other access point. The end of a day hike often brings hikers back to their starting point after completing a loop or going out and back along the same trail. However, it can also end at a different trailhead where prearranged transport awaits you.

Overnight, Multiday, or Long-Distance Hiking

As the name suggests, this type of hike involves one or more trails that take anything from two days to a few weeks to complete. Popular trails have shelters in place for hikers to overnight in. You may or may not be spending a few nights outside, so you'll be taking a few extra items of gear along, such as a sleeping bag, mattress, tent, a change of clothes, a lamp, and extra food and water.

Peak Bagging or Hill Bagging

Peak bagging is hiking with the goal of climbing or summiting a list of peaks or mountains in a specific area while on a hike. These peaks are often chosen based on their geographical location, significance, popularity, height, or view. Not only does completing the list give you bragging rights, but some peak-bagging clubs will give you an award for your accomplishment.

Backpacking

Backpacking involves a multiday hike with a backpack containing all your essential gear such as a tent, sleeping bag, food, cooking equipment, clothing, navigation tools, and first-aid supplies. The goal is to be self-sustained and able to set up camp anywhere if developed facilities aren't available.

Trekking

A trek is similar to a multiday or long-distance hike but with a few distinctions:

- A trek is more about reaching a specific destination than completing a trail.
- A trek can take you off the beaten path and into uncharted territory to reach that destination.

Thru-Hiking

Thru-hikes are not for the faint of heart. They refer to a few very long hikes with distinct endpoints that span distances of thousands of miles. They are completed in a single trip that may take a few weeks or many months to complete. The most well-known thru-hikes in the US are the Continental Divide Trail (CDT) which spans 3,100 miles, the Pacific Crest Trail (PCT) which is 2,700 miles, and the Appalachian Trail (AT) at 2,200 miles.

Glacier Hiking

Glacier hiking is seasonal and can only be done in the colder months when the ice is more stable. The terrain is inherently dangerous and can change at any time. Because of the increased risks, glacier hiking is best done in groups or with a guide. You will also need additional gear—on top of the usual setup—such as a helmet, ice axes, crampons, ropes, and suspender belts to name but a few.

Naked Hiking

No, it's not a joke. This is hiking wearing nothing but your hiking shoes and the pack on your back. It even has its own dedicated day, June 21st, otherwise known as the *summer solstice*. While it is more acceptable on this day, it's always a good idea to practice naked hiking on secluded trails where there is little to no risk of offending hikers who are not participating. Nudity is legal in national parks, as long as it's not sexual, but check the local and county laws before setting out in your birthday suit.

Choose a suitable trail and comfortable gear to avoid chafing and injury to your exposed skin. Use plenty of sunscreen, and be sure to take all your usual supplies along, including clothes.

Dog Hiking

This form of hiking involves taking your beloved pet along for the hike. You will need to take some extra gear along for your pup to have a good time as well, such as its food and water bowls, bed, harness or leash, and bags to pick up its poop, which contains bacteria that may be harmful to wildlife. The type of terrain and the wildlife in the area should also be considered, as your companion should be able to traverse it without being in danger.

Base Camping

Base camping involves setting up your campsite only once. From here, you can treat each day like an individual day hike or do other activities before returning to the comfort of the base camp every evening. It does, however, limit the distance you can travel on your hike, but it saves the time of setting up camp every day and takes the load of carrying your gear everywhere with you off your shoulders.

A BRIEF HISTORY OF HIKING

Hiking has been around for centuries, though its earliest practices were mainly out of necessity, exploration, or for ceremonial or religious reasons. Some of the oldest pilgrimages in the world are still popular today, such as El Camino de Santiago in Spain and Kumano Kodo in Japan, both of which are over a thousand years old and World Heritage Sites.

The earliest documented hikes date back to the end of the Middle Ages in 1334 and 1336 when French philosopher Jean Buridan and Italian scholar and poet Francesco Petrarca summited Mont Ventoux in southern France on separate occasions, the former for weather observations and the latter for recreation.

Before the mid-1700s there was no interest in hiking as it was seen as an activity for vagrants and drifters. This was quite the misconception, as a few decades later, hiking proved to require considerable resources in terms of finances, time, and effort. During the Romantic period of 1798–1837, hiking saw increased popularity as a recreational activity. Romantic thinkers, poets, and artists celebrated the untamed aspects of nature, embracing its wildness, sublimity, and mystery. They saw nature as a source of inspiration, awe, and emotional connection and encouraged a shift away from industrialization and urbanization. This sparked a renewed interest in exploring, conserving, and discovering the natural world.

During this time, many social clubs dedicated to hiking started popping up in the United States and it became a popular pastime for the most wealthy. It was only by the mid-1900s—after labor reform reduced working hours and gave workers paid time off—that hiking became more popular among the general population.

In the United Kingdom, the growing popularity of hiking was due in part to poets and authors who were avid hikers writing about their experiences and the people's need to escape from industrialization and urbanization. There was a slight problem though as much of the countryside was on private property, and access to it was therefore limited or prohibited. Nearly a century later, after decades of activism, the UK Parliament passed the National Parks and Access to the Countryside Act in 1949 which improved public access to natural areas and formed nationally protected lands.

In continental Europe, a greater appreciation for nature and the great outdoors was also kindled by 18th-century poets and authors who were inspired by the mountain ranges of the Germanic countries—most notably, the magnificent Alps. The Alps inspired not only writers but also early climbers, founding mountaineering and leading to greater interest in alpine ascents and exploration of other peaks worldwide.

Elsewhere in the world, recreational hiking became popular shortly after the Romantic period ended and was fueled mostly by expeditions and increased conservation efforts in the early to mid-1900s.

THE BENEFITS OF HIKING

Physical Fitness

Hiking works various muscle groups, particularly the lower body. Uphill climbs engage the glutes, quads, hamstrings, and calves, strengthening and toning these muscles. Descending slopes and navigating uneven terrain engage the stabilizing muscles, improving balance and coordination. Carrying a backpack during longer hikes also adds resistance and engages one's core, further enhancing muscle strength and endurance.

Hiking also involves a wide range of movements, such as stepping, climbing, jumping, and navigating obstacles, all of which improve joint mobility and flexibility. Varied and uneven terrain requires a greater range of motion, contributing to better flexibility in the hips, knees, ankles, and other joints.

Additionally, because hiking is a weight-bearing activity, it helps improve bone density. The impact of walking on uneven surfaces and the occasional jump stimulates bone growth and reduces the risk of osteoporosis. It also strengthens connective tissues and reduces the risk of fractures and injuries.

The physical benefits of hiking can vary depending on factors such as trail difficulty, duration, elevation gain, and individual fitness levels. Gradually increasing the intensity and duration of hikes over time can help maximize the physical fitness benefits while minimizing the risk of overexertion and injuries.

Mental Well-Being

Hiking has positive effects on mental health, which can indirectly benefit physical well-being. Spending time in nature, breathing fresh air, and being away from the stressors of everyday life can reduce anxiety, improve mood, and boost overall mental well-being. In short, it helps you get out of your head and observe the world around you.

Connection With Nature

Hiking offers an opportunity to practice mindfulness and connect with the present moment and the natural world that surrounds you. Walking amidst natural beauty encourages the mind to focus on your current experience—the sounds, sights, and scents of nature and the sensations you feel within the body. This mindfulness practice helps reduce rumination, increase self-awareness, and foster a deeper connection with oneself and the environment.

Fresh Air and Sunshine

Fresh air and sunshine have a positive impact on mood and mental health. The increased oxygen intake from fresh air stimulates the release of serotonin which promotes feelings of happiness and well-being. The higher concentration of oxygen in your blood supports cellular function, increases energy production, and invigorates the body. Sunlight also triggers the production of vitamin D, which is essential for maintaining healthy brain function and regulating mood.

The combination of physical activity, fresh air, sunlight, and natural surroundings during hiking can enhance vitality and leave you feeling more energized and refreshed.

Stress Relief

Hiking provides an opportunity to escape the hustle and bustle of daily life and immerse oneself in nature. Being surrounded by natural landscapes—such as forests, mountains, and rivers—can have a calming effect on the mind. The peacefulness and serenity of the outdoors—along with the combination of physical exertion, fresh air, and scenic beauty—create a positive environment that can enhance your mood and alleviate the symptoms of depression. Hiking releases endorphins that uplift your mood, reduce anxiety, and contribute to a sense of well-being.

Regular hiking can build your resilience to stress. Facing physical challenges, such as steep ascents or rough trails, and overcoming them enhances self-confidence and self-efficacy.

These qualities translate into everyday life, helping you cope with stressors more effectively and bounce back from adversity.

Social Interaction

Hiking as a group is an opportunity to build strong social connections. When people hike together, they share an extraordinary journey in nature, creating lasting memories and strengthening relationships. The act of hiking as a group encourages open communication and collaboration, as hikers work together to overcome challenges and navigate the trail. Hiking provides a sense of accomplishment as hikers achieve milestones together. The shared experiences and challenges encountered while hiking creates a unique opportunity to support and encourage each other.

Family hiking trips, in particular, offer numerous benefits. Parents and children can engage in shared experiences, cultivating a sense of unity and togetherness. It provides a platform to introduce children to the wonders of nature, encouraging curiosity and appreciation for the environment. As families tackle trails, they build resilience, teamwork, and problem-solving skills. They can plan routes together, decide on breaks and camp spots, and allocate responsibilities. These decisions foster a sense of responsibility and empower each family member to contribute to the journey.

Overall, hiking serves as a catalyst for social interaction and family bonding. By escaping into nature, putting aside distractions, and embracing shared experiences and challenges, hikers form deeper connections with one another and strengthen the bonds that tie people together.

Exploration and Adventure

Hiking offers you a unique opportunity to discover new things. Around every bend, there's a new sight to behold, whether it's a beautiful view of the landscape, a rare animal sighting, ancient ruins, an old cave, a hidden waterfall, you name it. The same trails can look drastically different depending on the season or even at different times of the day.

Improved Cognitive Function

Hiking stimulates the brain and improves cognitive function. Exposure to nature and changing surroundings enhances attention, concentration, and problem-solving abilities. It can also boost creativity and provide a mental break from daily routines, allowing the mind to rejuvenate and generate fresh ideas.

Heart Health

Hiking involves continuous movement and varying terrain, which help improve cardiovascular fitness. Uphill climbs and challenging trails increase heart rate, promoting a stronger heart and improved circulation. Regular hiking can enhance your endurance, allowing you to engage in more prolonged physical activities without fatigue.

Weight Management

Hiking is an effective way to burn calories and contribute to weight management. The varying intensity levels of hiking, including uphill climbs and rugged trails, increase calorie expenditure compared to walking on level surfaces. Regular hiking, combined with a healthy diet, can aid in weight loss or achieving weight-maintenance goals.

Improved Sleep

Engaging in regular hiking can establish a consistent sleep routine. By setting a regular schedule for hiking and maintaining physical activity during the day, your body becomes accustomed to a regular sleep-wake pattern. This helps regulate your internal body clock and promotes a more consistent and restful sleep each night.

The physically demanding nature of hiking engages various muscle groups and increases energy expenditure. The combination of cardiovascular exercise and muscular exertion helps to tire the body, making it easier to fall asleep at night. The more physically exhausted you are from hiking, the better your chances of experiencing deeper and more restful sleep.

Regular exposure to daylight during hiking can help reset your body's internal clock, promoting a healthy sleep-wake cycle. It helps synchronize your body's natural sleep-wake patterns, making it easier to fall asleep at night and wake up refreshed in the morning.

THINGS TO CONSIDER WHEN HIKING

Trail Difficulty

Before embarking on a hike, you should consider the trail's difficulty level. Factors such as distance, elevation gain, terrain, and the presence or absence of technical challenges determine the level of physical exertion and skill required. Longer distances demand endurance, while significant elevation gain tests strength and stamina. Terrain—whether flat and smooth or rugged and uneven—affects the need for balance and stability. Technical challenges like steep ascents, narrow paths, or rock scrambling demand agility and experience.

Weather Conditions

Checking the weather forecast beforehand and staying updated is essential as weather can sometimes change unexpectedly. Be prepared for these changes by packing the necessary gear to deal with them. Dressing appropriately, with layers, helps you adapt to temperature variations. Wearing moisture-wicking clothing and waterproof outer layers protects against rain and snow. Sunscreen, hats, and sunglasses protect against sun exposure. In challenging conditions, such as extreme heat or cold, adjusting plans or opting for safer trails may be necessary.

Trail Conditions

Stay aware and up-to-date on the trail conditions to ensure a safe and enjoyable experience. Pay attention to signs of muddy or slippery areas, which may require cautious footing. Be prepared for stream crossings by assessing water levels and finding stable crossing points. Watch out for potential hazards such as fallen trees, loose rocks, or overgrown vegetation that could impede progress or pose safety risks. Remaining vigilant and adapting to changing trail conditions helps prevent accidents and injuries. Sharing information about trail conditions with fellow hikers as you come across them contributes to a community of safety and support on the trails.

Navigation and Maps

Being knowledgeable about navigation techniques and having the right tools at hand minimizes the risk of getting lost, prevents you from being turned around, and saves valuable hiking time. Always carry a detailed map, compass, or GPS device to accurately navigate the trail. Familiarize yourself with the trail route beforehand, studying the landmarks, intersections, and potential points of confusion. Pay attention to trail markers, signs, or cairns (piles of stone markers) along the way. Use the map and compass to orient yourself and confirm your location. If using a GPS device, ensure it is fully charged and loaded with the necessary maps.

Safety Equipment

A well-stocked first-aid kit can address minor injuries and provide initial assistance in emergencies. A whistle can be used to signal for help if needed. A reliable headlamp or flashlight ensures visibility during low-light conditions. Ropes and gloves may also come in handy but aren't necessary for most trails.

For remote or challenging hikes, consider carrying a personal locator beacon (PLB) to alert rescue services in case of emergencies. These safety measures ensure preparedness and provide peace of mind, allowing you to handle unexpected situations effectively.

Physical Preparedness

Assess your fitness level honestly, and choose a trail that aligns with your abilities. It can be tempting to jump right into the deep end, but pace yourself. Starting with shorter or less challenging routes is wise for beginners. Take breaks along the way to rest and recover. Stay hydrated by carrying an adequate water supply and drinking regularly. Listen to your body's signals, and adjust your pace or difficulty level accordingly. Proper nutrition and snacks provide sustained energy. Engaging in regular exercise and strength training can improve endurance and prepare your body for the demands of hiking.

Leave No Trace

Adhering to the principles of *Leave No Trace* to protect the natural environment is a must. Pack up all trash, and dispose of it properly, leaving the trail and surrounding areas clean.

Respect wildlife by observing from a distance and not disturbing their natural behavior. Stay on designated trails to prevent damage to fragile ecosystems and vegetation. Avoid littering, excessive noise, or actions that may harm the environment. By practicing Leave No Trace, you help preserve the beauty of nature, keep the ecosystem in balance, and also ensure that others can enjoy the same unspoiled wilderness.

Wildlife Awareness

Be mindful of wildlife, and prioritize their safety and your own. Educate yourself about the local wildlife species, their habitats, and their behaviors. Understand how to safely encounter and coexist with them. Maintain a safe distance, and avoid approaching or feeding wild animals as it can disrupt their natural behavior and pose risks to yourself, the animals, and future hikers who may encounter them. Observe them from a distance, using binoculars or a zoom lens for a closer look. Preserve natural ecosystems, and help ensure the well-being of the animals that call them home.

Time Management

Plan your hike according to daylight hours, ensuring you have enough time to complete the trail or get to your campsite before nightfall. Stay conscious of your turnaround time so that you can return before darkness falls. Starting early in the day allows for more flexibility and mitigates potential issues or time constraints that may arise. Be aware of your hiking pace, and factor in rest breaks and any sightseeing along the way. Consider the trail's difficulty level and your fitness level when estimating the time needed. Prioritizing time management ensures a safer and more relaxed hiking experience, allowing you to fully enjoy the journey without feeling rushed or having to set up camp in the dark.

Hiking Partners

Consider hiking with a companion or in a group, as it enhances safety, provides support, and adds to the overall enjoyment. Choose your hiking partner carefully as they may not be as fit as you are, but be considerate of their limitations. Hiking with others helps ensure that someone is there to assist in case of emergencies or unexpected situations. It also allows for shared experiences, creating lasting memories, and fostering a sense of camaraderie.

WHERE PEOPLE HIKE

U.S. National Parks

Grand Canyon National Park

The 277-mile-long canyon in northwestern Arizona sports stunning views and a wide range of hiking opportunities within the park itself. The South Rim is very popular among tourists, so for a less crowded experience, it's best to visit the North Rim, which sees only 10% of the visitors to the park. The best months to visit the park are March and November as during spring and fall, you have a perfect blend of good weather and fewer people on the trail.

Yellowstone National Park

Encompassing parts of Wyoming, Montana and Idaho, Yellowstone is the second oldest national park in the world and the United States' first national park. Yellowstone is composed of 2.2 million acres of pristine wilderness with a distinctive landscape due to geothermal activity below the surface. With more than 10,000 hydrothermal features—of which 300 or more are geysers—a great deal of wildlife, and 900 miles of hiking trails, it is well worth the visit. The park is best visited in spring or fall when there are fewer tourists around, but take care as grizzly bears wake from hibernation in spring and can be less than pleasant.

Rocky Mountain National Park

This park has more than 355 miles of trails ranging from easy to advanced. It is located in north central Colorado. The best seasons to visit the Rockies are summer, fall, and spring, though higher elevations can have snow until mid-June. The weather and sights are at their peak during summer, but it's also peak hiking season, and trails will be busy. The best months to go if you want to avoid crowds are April and

November, and the best area with fewer people overall is the western side of the park.

Mount Rainier National Park

Mount Rainier National Park, in the state of Washington, features some of the best hikes in the US. Abundant wildlife and picturesque scenery such as wildflowers, waterfalls, rolling grasslands, and lakes make Mount Rainier a popular destination. There are plenty of day hikes, as well as the 93-mile-long Wonderland Trail. The trails are well-maintained and offer breathtaking views of the Mount Rainier volcano and surrounding hills every step of the way. The hiking season is relatively short and lasts from July to October.

Yosemite National Park

Home of the famous El Capitan and Half Dome in Yosemite Valley, eastern central California, Yosemite National Park is among the best places in the world to rock climb, but it also has amazing hiking trails. The park features amazing views of the granite cliffs and domes, alpine lakes, Giant Sequoia redwoods, and wildflowers, as well as Yosemite Falls—the tallest waterfall in North America. The best months to visit the park are between May and September, when the weather is good and trails, roads, and campgrounds are mostly accessible.

Great Smoky Mountains National Park

This park straddles North Carolina and Tennessee. With 150 official trails, the Great Smoky Mountains National Park's trails total over 800 miles that boast spectacular views in any season. With so many options, it can be daunting to pick a trail. However, choosing what sights you want to see and the distance you want to hike narrows down your options considerably. The Appalachian Trail runs through the park for 72 miles, and this offers a good chance to see what the AT is like before attempting the trail's full distance. The best months to visit for avoiding crowds are from March to May, though the weather is less than ideal.

Utah's "Mighty Five" National Parks

- **Arches National Park:** All 47 of the trails in Arches National Park are 7 miles or less and are easy to moderate in difficulty. The park is known for its thousands of red-rock arches and balancing rocks. It sees its busiest times from April to May and again in September and October. During its peak season, the park requires you to make a reservation to avoid disappointment.
- **Bryce Canyon National Park:** Not only does Bryce Canyon look amazing from above but also when viewed from below among the hoodoos (tall, thin spires of rock). The park's official trails are kept in good repair and are all relatively short, with

Fairyland Loop being the longest at 7.8 miles. This park can be visited all year round, with park services plowing and salting the road after each snowstorm. September is the best month to visit Bryce Canyon.

- **Canyonlands National Park:** There are more than 75 trails in the 527 square miles of the Canyonlands with spectacular sights that include the Mesa Arch, Horseshoe Canyon, and Confluence Overlook where the Green River and the Colorado River merge. The longest trail in Canyonlands is Shafer Trail at 183.3 miles. The best months to go to Canyonlands are April, May, September, and October when the weather is not too frigid or scorching. It is always smart to bring an extra layer of clothes as the temperatures of this high-altitude desert can change suddenly.

- **Capitol Reef National Park:** This park features the Waterpocket Fold, a 100-mile-long monocline—a literal fold in the surface of the Earth. Its sandstone canyons are similar to those found in Zion National Park, but Capitol Reef National Park has fewer tourists visiting. March to June and September to October are the best times to go to Capitol Reef because of the ideal weather conditions. As with the other parks in the region, be aware that temperatures can change suddenly.

- **Zion National Park:** The park covers 232 square miles and features a network of deep and narrow sandstone canyons, cliffs, and diverse plant and wildlife. The three most popular trails, Angel's Landing, The Subway, and The Narrows require a permit and possibly even timed reservations, so it's best to plan accordingly. The best months to visit Zion are April to May and September to October, when the weather is fair and the crowds are thinner.

Joshua Tree National Park

The Mojave and Colorado deserts meet in Joshua Tree, merging two unique ecosystems. This southern California park features a beautiful variety of plant and animal life, cultural history, and amazing geological features. There are over a hundred trails in the park, with a trail to suit almost everyone. This park is one of the best places in the US to go rock climbing. It is open all year round, but the best months to go are March to May and October to November, when the temperature and weather are ideal for hiking.

Death Valley National Park

Despite the name and its being a desert, Death Valley boasts a great variety of plant and animal life; it even has a set of three waterfalls called the Darwin Falls. The spring wildflowers are a phenomenal sight to see and bloom in late March and early April, making March one of the Park's busiest months. The best months to go to Death Valley are March to May and October to November, when the temperature and weather are ideal for hiking; the hot summer months should be avoided as the temperatures can soar to dangerous heights. The park also boasts some of the world's most ideal views of the sky, perfect for astrophotography and stargazing. The park has a lot of trails with varying difficulties to choose from. It straddles the Nevada-California border.

International Destinations

The Alps

One of the world's premier hiking destinations, this mountain range captivates outdoor enthusiasts with its breathtaking beauty and diverse landscapes. Stretching across several European countries, including France, Switzerland, Italy, Austria, and Germany, the Alps offer an extensive network of well-marked trails, catering to hikers of all skill levels. From gentle meadow walks to challenging alpine ascents, the region boasts a variety of routes with awe-inspiring views of snow-capped peaks, lush valleys, glacial lakes, and picturesque villages. Hikers are drawn to the Alps for its rich cultural heritage, pristine wilderness, and unforgettable experiences in nature.

Peru

Peru is a mesmerizing and enchanting hiking destination that beckons adventurers from around the globe. The country's diverse landscapes offer a plethora of trails to explore, including the world-renowned Inca Trail leading to the iconic Machu Picchu. Hikers can immerse themselves in the ancient history and culture of the Incas while traversing breathtaking mountain passes, lush cloud forests, and fascinating archaeological sites. Beyond Machu Picchu, Peru boasts lesser-known yet equally stunning routes like the Huayhuash Circuit and the Colca Canyon. With its rich history, vibrant culture, and awe-inspiring scenery, Peru offers a truly unforgettable and transformative hiking experience.

Nepal

Nepal stands as an unrivaled hiking destination, capturing the hearts of adventurers with its majestic Himalayan peaks, including the iconic Mount Everest. The country's diverse terrain offers an array of trekking options, from challenging high-altitude routes to serene trails through lush valleys and picturesque villages. The Annapurna Circuit, Langtang Valley, and Everest Base Camp are just a few of the popular trails that reveal Nepal's unique cultural heritage and breathtaking landscapes. The warmth and hospitality of the Nepalese people add to the allure, making Nepal a must-visit destination for hikers seeking both physical challenges and spiritual enrichment amidst some of the world's most awe-inspiring scenery.

Iceland

Known as the "Land of Fire and Ice," Iceland calls to hikers with its otherworldly landscapes and raw, untouched beauty. This Nordic isl and boasts a diverse array of hiking trails, ranging from lava fields to glaciers, waterfalls, geysers, and rugged coastlines. The famous Laugavegur and Fimmvörðuháls trails offer mesmerizing views of multicolored mountains and hot springs. Exploring Iceland's pristine wilderness provides an unparalleled connection to nature, where hikers can witness the forces of geothermal activity and marvel at its untamed wilderness. With its unique blend of natural wonders and geological marvels, Iceland presents an unforgettable and adventurous experience for hikers of all skill levels.

Patagonia

This breathtaking region at the southern tip of South America lures hikers with its dramatic landscapes and wilderness. Towering granite peaks, sprawling glaciers, turquoise lakes, and vast grasslands create a surreal backdrop for unforgettable hiking experiences. Iconic trails like the Torres del Paine Circuit and the Fitz Roy Trek beckon adventurers seeking a true communion with nature. Patagonia's diverse terrain offers challenges and rewards, from thrilling ascents to tranquil valleys. Hikers can encounter unique wildlife while immersing themselves in the region's rich cultural heritage.

The Canadian Rockies

The Canadian Rockies stand as an enchanting haven for hikers, boasting awe-inspiring vistas and a wealth of outdoor adventures. Nestled in western Canada, this vast mountain range offers an array of trails catering to all skill levels. From leisurely strolls by emerald lakes to challenging alpine ascents, the Rockies present a diverse landscape of rugged peaks, dense forests, and cascading waterfalls. Hikers can revel in encounters with wildlife, including elk and mountain goats. With their untouched wilderness and picturesque beauty, the Canadian Rockies beckon explorers seeking to reconnect with nature and forge unforgettable memories amid the majesty of the great outdoors.

The Drakensberg Mountains

Bordering South Africa and Lesotho, this mountain range is a hiker's paradise, offering a breathtaking blend of rugged terrain and striking beauty. This World Heritage Site entices adventurers with its stunning landscapes, including dramatic cliffs, lush valleys, and cascading waterfalls. The extensive network of trails caters to hikers of all skill levels, from leisurely day hikes to challenging multiday treks. Hikers can immerse themselves in the region's rich biodiversity, spotting rare flora and fauna along the way. The Drakensberg's cultural significance is also evident in its ancient rock art sites, providing a unique and enriching experience for nature enthusiasts and history buffs alike.

FINDING A HIKING TRAIL NEAR YOU

There are plenty of resources available online to help you find hiking trails near you. Here are a few to help you scout out the perfect hike:

- **Alltrails:** A website with a vast database of hiking trails worldwide, providing trail information, reviews, ratings, photos, and difficulty levels.
- **TrailLink by Rails-to-Trails:** An app that covers over 40,000 miles of trails, offering reviews, photos, and the ability to track favorite trails.
- **Trailforks:** A map-based app primarily designed for mountain bikers but useful for hikers as well, with crowd-sourced trail information and maps.
- **Yelp:** A review site that provides recommendations and reviews for hiking trails, including specific requests such as waterfalls or dog-friendly trails.
- **TripAdvisor:** A resource with information and reviews about popular hikes worldwide, along with suggestions for accommodations and activities.
- **National Forests, National Park Service, and State Park Sites:** Visit the websites of these government organizations for basic information on hiking trails, including length and difficulty.
- **Local Trail Websites:** Some areas have websites or community organizations dedicated to hiking and

outdoor exploration, providing information on local trails.

- **Social Media Hashtags:** Explore hashtags related to hiking in your city or area on platforms like Instagram to find posts and recommendations from locals.
- **Search Engine Queries:** Use search engines like Google, YouTube, and Pinterest to find lists, videos, and articles about the best hiking trails in specific locations.
- **Local Municipal and State Government Sites:** Check the "Parks and Recreation" pages of local government websites for information on hiking trails in the area.

Don't like searching for a trail online? Try the old-fashioned way:

- Outdoor Retailers: Retailers like REI, Patagonia, and Eastern Mountain Sports offer content on outdoor activities and often sponsor hiking clubs or events. Strike up a conversation with the salespeople at outdoor retailers as many of them are outdoor enthusiasts themselves.
- Talk to other hikers you meet on the trail. Nothing beats learning about a trail from someone who has experienced it.

- Your neighbors and local friends can be a valuable resource for discovering nearby hiking trails that may be hidden gems. Reach out to friends or acquaintances in the area you plan to visit for recommendations and tips on finding local hiking trails.

SUMMARY

- Hiking is a centuries-old practice enjoyed by many who wish to escape into nature.
- There are various forms of hiking you can choose from to suit your outdoor lifestyle.
- National parks have some of the most astounding trails.
- Hiking offers a wealth of physical and mental health benefits.
- Careful consideration and planning of your hiking trip are essential for your safety and for you to have an enjoyable experience.
- Online as well as local resources are a wellspring of information to find trails near you.

Using what you've learned in this chapter, you can begin to assess your motives for hiking: whether you would like to get more active, break away from the urban environment, or experience the beauty of the natural world firsthand. Set yourself a few goals for what you would like to gain from your hiking trip, and choose a trail that serves your needs.

Now that you have learned what hiking is, how it originated as a recreational activity, its health benefits, and how to find the perfect trail, I'm sure you are eager to break away and experience the benefits the real world has to offer out on the trail.

It's almost time to get out there, but first, we'll look at some of the gear you will need before embarking on your hiking trip.

2

GEARING UP

Having the right gear makes the wilderness a playground, not a battlefield.

— UNKNOWN

THE RIGHT CLOTHES

C hoosing the right clothes for hiking is not only important for comfort but also for function as appropriate fabrics and layering regulate temperature, provide protection from the elements, and reduce the risk of injuries or discomfort, enhancing overall safety on the trail. The following is a list of do's and don'ts when it comes to your hiking attire:

- When choosing hiking pants, prioritize comfort and flexibility. Opt for pants made of moisture-wicking material to keep you dry and comfortable throughout your hike. Look for designs that offer ample freedom of movement, such as those with stretch or articulated knees. Well-fitting, comfortable pants will allow you to navigate the trail with ease and enhance your overall hiking experience.
- When selecting a hiking top, prioritize moisture-wicking fabrics that wick sweat away from the body and enhance evaporation to keep you cool and dry on the trail. You'll be thankful you did during those hot summer days. Also, look for tops with breathable mesh panels or ventilation features to enhance airflow and regulate body temperature, thus preventing you from overheating during your hike. Choose between short-sleeve or long-sleeve options based on weather conditions and personal preference, keeping in mind that long-sleeve shirts provide added sun protection and can be rolled up if needed.
- When preparing for colder conditions, make sure to pack a warm jacket for your hike. Consider options like a polyester fleece jacket or a puffy jacket with

polyester fill, as they provide insulation and retain heat effectively. These jackets offer warmth without adding excessive weight or bulk to your backpack. Layer the jacket over your base and mid-layers for added insulation during chilly weather. Having a warm jacket on hand ensures that you stay comfortable and protected from the cold, even if it sneaks up on you.

- A waterproof and breathable (yes, they can be both) rain jacket is a must-have for hiking in wet or potentially wet conditions. It keeps you dry by repelling rainwater while allowing moisture from sweat to escape, preventing that clammy feeling, keeping you comfortable, and allowing you to focus on the trail. Look for jackets with sealed seams and adjustable hoods to provide full protection.

- Wearing a brimmed hat while hiking serves multiple purposes. It shields your head, face, ears, and neck from both rain and sun, providing protection against harmful UV rays and keeping you dry during showers. Don't forget to wear sunglasses to safeguard your eyes from glare and potential eye strain, especially if you're likely to encounter patches of snow on the trail. These simple accessories contribute to your overall comfort, eye safety, and protection against the elements.

- A good pair of hiking shoes is perhaps the *most* important item you will have with you on your hike.

When choosing hiking footwear, prioritize sturdy shoes or boots that offer ankle support, protection, and traction. Only choose sandals for even terrain, as they don't provide much grip or ankle support on rougher terrain. Look for designs with durable construction, protective toe caps, and rugged outsoles for stability on different terrains. Proper ankle support reduces the risk of sprains. Ensure a good fit, and consider waterproof options for wet conditions. High-quality hiking footwear provides comfort, prevents foot fatigue, and has superior grip.

To ensure comfort and safety, it's best to avoid wearing the following items on a hike:

- **Clothes made of cotton or denim:** These materials have a tendency to absorb moisture, whether from sweat or rain, which can leave you feeling damp and uncomfortable. Once wet, cotton and denim can take a long time to dry and can potentially lead to chills or hypothermia in colder conditions. Instead, choose moisture-wicking and quick-drying fabrics—like synthetic blends or merino wool—that help regulate body temperature.
- **Clothes that you don't want to get dirty or ruined:** The trail environment can be rough and unpredictable, with potential encounters with mud, dust, branches, or other elements that may soil or

damage your clothing. Opt for clothing that is durable, easy to clean, and designed for outdoor activities.

- **Inappropriate or brand-new shoes:** Avoiding these is especially vital when embarking on longer hikes. Flip-flops won't cut it. Proper hiking shoes or boots that are broken in and have been tested on walks around the neighborhood or shorter hikes provide better support and reduce the risk of discomfort. Brand-new shoes can be stiff and may not conform to your feet properly, leading to painful rubbing or blisters. Opting for well-fitted, broken-in footwear ensures optimal comfort and minimizes the chance of unnecessary pain.

- **Jewelry:** Leaving jewelry at home is a wise decision to mitigate the risk of loss. Jewelry can easily become lost or damaged during outdoor activities due to the physical demands of hiking or potential snags on branches or rocks. Also, wearing jewelry increases the risk of injury as it can get caught on objects or pose a safety hazard in case of a fall.

BASIC HIKING GEAR

The 10 Essentials

Having the right gear for a hiking adventure can turn what would otherwise be an awful slog into a safe and enjoyable experience. The 10 Essentials are a list of gear recommended for hikes of any duration. They will enable you to respond properly to an emergency and prepare you for spending a safe night outdoors even when you didn't plan on it:

- navigational equipment, such as a compass, maps, or a GPS device
- sun protection, such as sunscreen, a hat, and sunglasses
- clothing suited to any conditions you may encounter on the hike based on the season, weather, altitude, and temperature
- a headlamp or flashlight and extra batteries
- first-aid supplies
- a knife
- fire starters
- emergency shelter
- food
- water

The following list provides an overview of basic hiking gear, including the 10 Essentials that will help you have a successful hike.

- A large, sturdy backpack allows you to carry all your gear, food, and water comfortably and efficiently. Look for a backpack with durable construction, adjustable straps, and multiple compartments for organized storage. Consider the size based on the duration and difficulty of your hikes. A well-packed backpack should distribute weight evenly across your back and onto your hips to reduce strain on your shoulders. Your gear should be secure and easily accessible. Smaller backpacks, like day packs, are convenient for carrying the 10 Essentials on a day hike.

- Dependable hiking boots or shoes with good traction for any type of hike.
- Invest in a good pair of moisture-wicking socks to keep your feet comfortable and dry during any type of hike. These specialized socks are designed to pull moisture away from the skin, promoting evaporation and reducing the risk of excessive sweating. By keeping your feet dry, moisture-wicking socks minimize the chances of friction and hotspots, which can lead to painful blisters. Look for socks made of synthetic or merino wool materials as they have excellent moisture-wicking properties.
- Navigation tools such as a map, compass, and GPS device are essential for route finding during a hike of any kind. A detailed map provides valuable information about the trail, landmarks, and potential hazards. A compass helps determine direction and maintain orientation. A GPS device offers precise location tracking and additional navigational features. Carrying these tools ensures you can confidently navigate the trail, make informed

decisions, and avoid getting lost. Familiarize yourself with their usage beforehand to effectively utilize these navigation tools.

- A headlamp or flashlight is a vital piece of gear for any hiking adventure, particularly for navigating in low-light conditions or during emergencies. It provides illumination and enhances visibility on the trail, ensuring safe movement in the dark. A hands-free headlamp allows you to have full use of your hands for balance and other tasks, especially when nature calls in the dead of night. In case of unexpected situations or delays, a headlamp or flashlight becomes invaluable for extending your hiking time and finding your way back to safety. A headlamp comes in handy for multiday hikes or for starting a day hike before dawn or finishing it after sunset.

- Bring extra clothing layers for adapting to changing weather conditions during a hike. Depending on the forecast, pack additional layers that offer warmth or protection against rain. Consider packing gloves and a spare pair of socks for added comfort. This is particularly essential for multiday hikes.

- A waterproof jacket and pants create a barrier against moisture, preventing water from seeping through and drenching your clothes. You may need to bring a waterproof jacket along on your day hike if the weather is likely to change, but it's essential for a multiday hike.

- A brimmed hat and sunglasses protect your head and eyes and are must-haves for both day hikes and multiday hikes.
- Sunscreen and insect repellent are necessary items for hiking. Sunscreen with a high SPF protects your skin from harmful UV rays, reducing the risk of sunburn and long-term skin damage. Insect repellent keeps pesky bugs at bay, preventing bites and potential diseases. First, apply sunscreen generously and reapply as needed, then use insect repellent according to the instructions. Pest repellent and sunscreen are a must for any type of hike, even when the weather is overcast.
- A water bottle or hydration system is a necessity for hikes of any duration. Staying hydrated is crucial for maintaining energy, preventing dehydration, and optimizing physical performance. Choose a water bottle or hydration system that is lightweight, durable, and easy to carry. Natural water sources may be scarce or nonexistent. Consider the length and intensity of your hike and pack enough water to last the duration, accounting for the weather, availability of water along the trail, and exertion level. Regularly sip from your water source to stay hydrated and replenish fluids as needed.

- Packing snacks and food is vital for maintaining energy levels and sustenance during a hike. The more intense the hike, the more energy you will burn and the more you will need to eat. Opt for lightweight, high-energy snacks such as trail mix, energy bars, dried fruits, or nuts. These provide quick and easily accessible sources of nutrients and calories. Pack lightweight or dehydrated meals that are easy to prepare and consume on the trail, such as sandwiches or prepackaged meals. Having a variety of snacks and food ensures that you don't get bored with your options and have fuel to sustain your body throughout the hike. Pack at least a snack for a day hike and be sure to take enough food and snacks along on a multiday hike.

- Carrying a first-aid kit is absolutely essential when hiking any length of trail as it provides basic medical supplies to treat minor injuries you may sustain on the way. It should include adhesive bandages, antiseptic wipes, gauze pads, adhesive tape, tweezers, and pain relievers. Also consider including items like blister pads, insect bite ointment, and any necessary personal medications. A well-stocked first-aid kit enables you to handle cuts, scrapes, blisters, and other minor ailments promptly, ensuring your safety and well-being on the trail. Regularly check and replenish your kit to keep it up to date and ready for any unexpected situations.

Injuries can occur on any trail, so take a first-aid kit along on every hike.

- Carry an emergency whistle. In case of emergencies or if you need to signal for help, a loud whistle can attract attention from a distance. Whistles are lightweight, compact, and highly effective at cutting through ambient noise. They can be heard over long distances, even in dense forests or during inclement weather. Having an emergency whistle as part of your gear enhances your safety and increases the chances of being located and assisted quickly in critical situations. A whistle is lightweight and should be carried along on any type of hike.

- Carrying a multi-tool or pocket knife comes in handy while hiking, as it serves a multitude of purposes and can be indispensable in emergency situations. These versatile tools typically include features such as blades, screwdrivers, scissors, can openers, and more. They can be used for tasks like cutting, opening packages, repairing gear, or preparing food. In emergencies, a multi-tool or pocket knife can assist with first aid, building shelters, and making essential repairs to other gear. A good knife can even save your life during encounters with aggressive wildlife. Having a sharp tool readily available adds to your self-sufficiency and preparedness on the trail, so it's a good idea to carry one along on any type of hike.

- Include personal hygiene items in your hiking gear for maintaining cleanliness and comfort on the trail. Pack essentials such as toilet paper, hand sanitizer, biodegradable soap, and other hygiene items. Toilet paper ensures hygiene during bathroom breaks, while hand sanitizer helps keep hands clean when access to water is limited. Biodegradable soap allows you to practice Leave No Trace principles when washing dishes or cleaning yourself. It's good to have hygiene items on a day hike in case nature calls unexpectedly, but it certainly is necessary for a multiday hike.

- Carrying extra batteries or a solar-powered charger is essential if you rely on electronic devices during your hike. Whether it's for a GPS device, headlamp, or other battery-powered items, having spare batteries ensures uninterrupted functionality. Check the compatibility and power requirements of your devices to pack the appropriate spares. In remote areas or longer hikes, access to new batteries may be limited, so extras will come in handy. It's not essential for a day hike, but it certainly is for a multiday hike or whenever you are using a GPS device.

- Carrying an emergency shelter—such as a lightweight tarp or emergency bivouac—is important to have for unexpected situations while hiking.

These shelters provide protection from the elements and help maintain body heat if you're caught in adverse conditions or forced to spend an unexpected night outdoors. Lightweight and compact, they can be easily packed in your backpack as a precautionary measure. Having an emergency shelter ensures you're prepared for unforeseen circumstances, providing a sense of security and increasing your chances of weathering unexpected situations safely. It's an essential item for a day or multiday hike.

- A trekking or camping stove is a valuable item for outdoor enthusiasts, providing the means to cook meals and boil water on the trail. These compact and portable stoves are designed for efficiency and convenience, allowing you to prepare hot meals and beverages. They use various fuel sources such as gas canisters or liquid fuel, and some models offer adjustable heat control for versatile cooking options. A stove is not necessary for a day hike, but it is indispensable for hot meals on a multiday hike.

- Bring lightweight and compact cookware and utensils for preparing your meals while hiking for several days. Opt for lightweight pots, pans, and dishes made of durable materials like aluminum or titanium. Look for collapsible or nesting designs to save space in your backpack. Include lightweight utensils such as a spoon, fork, and knife. These are not required items for day hikes, but they are for multiday hikes.

- Carrying a water purification method is crucial for accessing safe drinking water from natural sources while day hiking in hot weather or for multiday hiking. Options include water filters, purifiers, or water treatment tablets. These methods effectively remove or neutralize contaminants, bacteria, and parasites, ensuring the water is safe to consume. Choose a lightweight purification method that suits your needs. Be sure to check the availability of water sources along your route. Having a reliable water purification system allows you to stay well hydrated, even when natural water sources are your only option.

- A trekking or camping tent is a necessity for multiday hikes. These shelters provide protection from the elements, privacy, and a comfortable place to rest and sleep. Look for lightweight and compact designs that are easy to set up and pack, especially if you'll be doing so for several days. Consider the size of the tent based on the number of occupants and the conditions you expect to encounter.

- A sleeping bag and sleeping pad or mattress are vital for multiday hikes. A sleeping bag provides warmth and insulation, keeping you comfortable throughout the night. Look for a bag with a temperature rating suitable for the conditions you'll encounter. A sleeping pad or mattress offers cushioning and insulation from the ground, enhancing overall comfort and helping to regulate body temperature. Together, a quality sleeping bag and pad ensure a restful night's sleep.

- Garbage bags are great for ensuring responsible waste management and leaving no trace behind. Pack lightweight and durable bags to pack up your trash and keep the trail clean. Properly disposing of waste prevents littering, protects wildlife, and maintains the natural beauty of the environment. Remember to tidy up not only your own trash but also other litter you encounter. By doing this, you contribute to preserving the pristine condition of the trail for future hikers to enjoy. Garbage bags are needed for multiday hikes.

TREKKING POLES: WHAT ARE THEY AND DO YOU NEED THEM?

Trekking poles, sometimes called hiking poles, are carbon fiber or aluminum shafts with a handle on one end and a sharp point or grip on the other. They can be used singly, like a staff, or as a pair to help give you stability on trails and uneven terrain. Using two trekking poles instead of a hiking staff offers you better balance and traction and is the preferred option for most hikers. Trekking poles aren't a necessity for hiking, but they can make hiking a lot easier. Let's look at some of the benefits of using trekking poles:

- They give you extra stability when ascending or descending. You may need to adjust the length of your trekking poles for comfort and stability when going uphill or downhill—an inch or two shorter for uphills and an inch or two longer for downhills—but it depends on personal preference. Most hikers don't bother adjusting their poles once they are at the standard length for their height.
- They are great at reducing knee strain when descending. This is especially helpful when you are carrying a heavy backpack. Instead of your knees taking all the strain, trekking poles transfer some of the energy from impacts to your upper body. By engaging your upper body, you'll also get more of a full-body workout from your hike.
- Trekking poles provide you with better balance on rough terrain or while crossing rivers by giving you more points of contact with the terrain beneath you. This enables you to navigate obstacles faster and with greater confidence.
- They can double as tent poles. Freestanding tents are heavier than non-freestanding tents due to the tent poles that they come with, so by switching to a non-freestanding tent or a tarp, you cut down on nearly a pound of your gear's weight.

- By using trekking poles, you naturally develop a rhythm while walking. This makes it easier to keep moving at a certain pace as you tend to avoid breaking the rhythm by changing pace, thus making you hike just a little bit faster.
- You can use trekking poles to push tree branches or a poisonous plant's foliage out of the way safely without having to touch them with your hands.
- You can use trekking poles as probes to test the depth of the water or mud when crossing murky streams and rivers. Also, when the terrain is obscured by snow or ice you can test the depth of the snow or the strength of the ice to ensure a safer crossing.
- Trekking poles offer greater traction on wet or slippery terrain, making them especially useful in wet or rainy weather.
- You can use trekking poles as a last resort to fend off wild animals in the event of a bad encounter by banging them together or raising them into the air to appear bigger. They may even prove useful for defense when things get physical.
- Trekking poles can reduce fatigue when carrying a heavy backpack or when hiking long-distance on multiday trails.
- If you are one of the unlucky people whose hands swell while ascending, using trekking poles will

reduce the swelling and discomfort by raising your hands closer to the level of your heart.

There is quite a range of trekking poles on the market, which can make choosing the right pair difficult. Next, we'll highlight some of the features trekking poles have to help narrow down your choices:

- Trekking poles are sold as pairs and often have grips or straps that are right- and left-hand specific.
- Trekking poles are usually made of aluminum or carbon fiber. While carbon fiber poles are lighter and more shock absorbent, they can snap if handled too roughly. Aluminum poles are slightly heavier but more durable.
- Some trekking poles have built-in shock absorbers. While not completely necessary, they might add a little bit more comfort.
- Trekking poles have a variety of grip materials:
- Cork: Best for hot-weather hikes, these grips resist moisture and provide a good grip even when your hands are sweaty. They also absorb some shock.
- Foam: These grips are soft, comfortable, shock-absorbent, and they absorb sweat.
- Rubber: Best for cold-weather hikes, they insulate your hands and provide shock absorption. Their downside is that they can chafe or cause blisters on sweaty hands.

- Plastic: Avoid hard plastic grips, even if they are molded, as your hands are likely to slip on them or chafe and blister.
- The general rule when choosing the correct length of trekking poles is to hold the pole like you would hold it when hiking with the tip on the ground. Your arm should form a 90-degree angle at your elbow when the pole is the right length. Some trekking poles aren't adjustable, so here's a quick guide to choosing the correct length:
- If you are 5 ft or shorter, you'll need a maximum pole length of 39 in.
- For 5 ft 1 in.–5 ft 7 in., a maximum pole length of 43 in.
- For 5 ft 8 in.–5 ft 11 in., a maximum pole length of 47 in.
- And if you're over 6 ft, you'll need a maximum pole length of 51 in.
- Trekking poles with adjustable lengths will either collapse telescopically or fold up for easy storage. Telescopic trekking poles are easily adjustable and great for getting the perfect fit for whatever terrain you're hiking on. Because they have more parts, they are a little heavier than fixed-length trekking poles.
- Adjustable trekking poles will have either a twist-lock or clip-lock system to secure them at their desired lengths. Clip-locks are the better choice as twist-lock systems tend to wear out over time and

slip, which can compromise your stability when leaning on them.

Remember that trekking poles and hiking staffs are not substitutes for medical canes for urban use.

WHAT TO DO IF YOU FORGET YOUR GEAR

We've likely all felt that awful feeling halfway into a trip when you realize you forgot something important at home. That feeling is much, much worse when you're in the wilderness, miles away from civilization. It happens to the best of us. Though there's a workaround for some situations, others may require you to cut your hike short and turn back. Here are a few examples of commonly forgotten gear and what you can do about your situation if it happens to you.

Tent Poles

- All is not lost yet. You can improvise by propping your tent up using trekking poles, a camera tripod, a spare pole from a hiking companion, or even a rigid branch. Your tent will be noticeably saggy, but it should do.
- Another method is to use some cordage to suspend the top of the tent up off the ground:

1. Find a suitable spot between two trees or boulders to which you can securely tie the ends of the cordage.

2. Tie the cordage down at a height equal to or slightly above that of your tent.
3. Run it across the top of your tent, and tie the cordage down opposite but at the same height as the first.
4. Tie the tent's pole sleeves or clips to the suspended line.
5. Stake the corners of the tent down.

- You won't always be guaranteed to have convenient trees or boulders nearby to tie the cordage to. If all else fails and the weather and insects permit it, you can cowboy camp under the stars, and if the ground is wet, you can use the flattened body of your tent as a tarp underneath your sleeping bag.
- Natural shelters like caves, rock overhangs, fallen trees, or dense, low-hanging branches can also be used as shelters.
- If the weather looks stormy and you are able to turn back, you should, but most of the time, you'll only notice the missing poles once you're setting up camp and have little daylight left. In this case, it might be necessary to build a survival shelter for the night.

Sleeping Bag

- The easiest option is to share a sleeping bag with a friend. Zip a sleeping bag open, and use it as a blanket to sleep under together. You might need to wear additional layers or headwear to stay warm.

- If you're on your own and you have a bivouac sack or an emergency blanket, either will do the trick, provided the weather isn't too cold.
- If the weather is cold enough to risk hypothermia, you'll need to turn back.

Sleeping Pad or Mattress

- It's possible to go without a sleeping pad in fair weather. Find a smooth flat surface to pitch your tent.
- You can improvise by using extra clothing or a backpack as a sleeping pad. Though it won't be comfortable, it will help insulate you from the cold ground.
- If the ground is covered by snow or the weather is cold enough to risk hypothermia, you'll need to turn back.

Hiking Shoes

Luckily, you'll know that you forgot your hiking footwear before you even begin the hike. Though, in most situations, there's no way around forgetting your hiking footwear, you can still continue if the trail is dry, hard-packed, and even.

You'll need to turn back in the event of any of the following:

- You only have flip-flops or shoes with no back.
- Your shoes are not waterproof, and the trail is wet.
- The terrain is rough, slippery, or uneven.
- Your shoes are not sturdy, they don't have good tread or are likely to put you at risk of injury.
- Your shoes are uncomfortable and likely to give you blisters.

Water Filter

A forgotten water filter doesn't have to mean the end of your trip. You can filter debris out of a natural water source using an item of clothing and then bring it to a rolling boil for one minute—three minutes if you are at or above an elevation of 6,500 ft. Once cool, the water is safe to drink, or you can pour it into your bottle.

Although not advised, you can drink water directly from a fast-moving stream, but you risk ingesting parasites like *Giardia*.

Stove

Forgetting your stove also doesn't mean the end of your trip, unless you didn't bring any dehydrated food along. Dehydrated camping meals can be soaked in cold water until they are soft. This might take anything from a few minutes to over an hour, depending on the type of food. Make sure to periodically test the food to see if it's softened up enough to be palatable. It won't be the best meal you've ever had, but it will sustain you.

Headlamp

If you forgot your headlamp, you can use your phone's flashlight in a pinch, although it's not recommended. It should work fine around the campsite, but it's not bright enough to hike with and will quickly drain the battery. Instead, make as much use of the available daylight as possible by setting out before daybreak and finishing the day's hike and dinner before nightfall. You'll need to turn back if you were planning on setting up camp anywhere it would be dangerous to move about in the dark, like near fast-flowing rivers or dangerous drops.

SUMMARY

- Check the weather to make sure you bring appropriate clothing on your hike.
- Hike only with reliable hiking footwear.
- Always carry a first-aid kit. Injuries can happen at any time.
- Always carry an emergency shelter and blanket with you.
- Decide if investing in a pair of trekking poles is for you.

- Forgetting an essential piece of gear doesn't spell the end of your hiking trip. For some things, there are workarounds.

DAY HIKING PACKING CHECKLIST

- daypack
- appropriate clothing for the weather
- hiking footwear
- enough food and snacks (beyond minimum expectation)
- enough water (beyond minimum expectation)
- navigation tools (maps, compass, GPS device)
- first-aid kit
- multi-tool or knife
- sun protection (sunglasses, hat, sunscreen)
- fire
- emergency bivouac or tarp

BACKPACKING CHECKLIST

Backpacking Gear

- backpack
- backpacking tent
- sleeping bag
- headlamp

Clothing

- moisture-wicking underwear
- moisture-wicking T-shirts
- quick-drying pants
- long-sleeve shirts (for sun and bugs)
- lightweight fleece or jacket
- boots or shoes suited to the terrain
- socks
- extra clothes

Additional Clothing for Rainy and Cold Weather

- rain jacket and pants
- long underwear
- warm insulated jacket or vest
- fleece pants
- gloves
- warm hat

Camp Kitchen

- backpacking stove
- fuel
- cookware
- dishes or bowls
- eating utensils
- mugs or cups

- biodegradable soap
- small towel
- water container
- bear canister, food sack, or hang bag with 50 ft cord
- lighter or matches (in waterproof container)

Navigation

- map
- compass
- GPS device

Food and Water

- water bottle
- water filter
- meals
- snacks
- drinks
- extra food (beyond minimum expectation)

Health and Hygiene

- hand sanitizer
- toothbrush and toothpaste
- sanitation trowel
- toilet paper or wipes and a sealable bag (to pack it up)

- menstrual products
- prescription medications
- prescription glasses
- sunglasses (and retainer leash)
- sunscreen
- SPF-rated lip balm
- sun hat

Tools and Repair Kits

- multi-tool or knife
- puncture repair kit for mattress
- sewing kit
- duct tape

Emergency Items

- first-aid kit
- whistle
- fire starters
- emergency shelter
- itinerary to be left with a friend
- itinerary to be left in the vehicle

Personal Items

- permits
- passport

- credit card or cash
- identification
- car keys
- cellphone

Now that you have learned about the different items of gear you will need on your hike, how to use them to spend time outdoors, and how to make do without them in a pinch, you are on the threshold of the great outdoors.

In the following chapter, you will learn how to avoid getting lost by knowing your way around a topographical map and learning how to navigate using a compass.

3

NAVIGATION STATION

The art of navigation is knowing where you are while never losing sight of where you're heading.

— UNKNOWN

HOW TO USE A MAP

E ven though GPS devices can tell you where you are with great accuracy, they sometimes still experience interference from cliffs or densely forested areas. Relying solely on technology for your hike can be problematic, especially if the battery runs out, your device malfunctions, or you lose it.

Navigating the wilderness confidently begins with the fundamental skill of map reading. We will now delve into the art of deciphering maps and unlocking the secrets they hold for successful navigation. From understanding symbols and contour lines to plotting routes, I will guide you through the techniques and knowledge needed to navigate the trails using traditional paper maps.

Choose the Right Type of Map

Not every type of map will do on a hike; for instance, tourist maps are often not to scale and lack several crucial features necessary for hiking, and road maps—though they are to scale and feature details of man-made structures and rivers —are not very helpful either.

The best maps for hikers to have are topographical maps due to their detailed representation of the terrain and elevation changes. Unlike regular maps, topographical maps show contour lines that allow hikers to understand the steepness of slopes and identify features like ridges, valleys, and peaks. This valuable information helps hikers plan routes, antici-pate challenges, and make informed decisions based on the landscape.

Choose the Right Scale

Consider the scale of the map and if it applies to the type of activity you will be doing. A map with a large scale will show more details of a smaller area and is great when covering short distances, like when day hiking or for short trails. A map with a small scale shows fewer details of a larger area and is great when you'll be covering a lot of distance, like during multiday hikes, long trail runs, or cycling.

For example, on a smaller, 1:25,000 scale map, 1 cm of the map represents 250 m in reality and the grid squares are 4 cm X 4 cm, representing 1 km². On a larger, 1:50,000 scale map, 1 cm of the map represents 500 m in reality and the grid squares are 2 cm X 2 cm, representing 1 km².

Understanding Map Symbols and Their Meanings

Maps can seem chaotic and daunting initially, and to further complicate things, not all map brands use the same symbols and color codes. However, the truth is that reading a map is easier than it seems, provided you consult the legend. The legend, also known as the key, appears in the corner of the map and contains the various symbols and lines used and their meanings. It's a good idea to familiarize yourself with the map brand you are using so that interpreting it will be easy.

The paths that are most useful to hikers are the ones that indicate a public right of way. These will include trails that you can walk or ride along using a horse or bicycle. As is often the case, a path indicated on the map may not be as obvious in reality. It could have become overgrown or been rerouted. Also, many unofficial paths and trails might not be indicated on the map, so periodically check your map and surroundings for indicated landmarks to ensure you are still on the right track.

Maps may distinguish between the types of trees growing in a wooded area by using icons shaped like the trees found there. This can be a helpful landmark to help you navigate an area.

Contour Lines

Contour lines represent the elevation and shape of the land. These curved, meandering lines connect points of equal height above a reference point, typically sea level. By understanding contour lines, you can visualize the steepness of terrain, valleys, and ridges. To identify contour lines on a map, look for lines that form closed loops, indicating hills or mountains. Concentric lines represent elevation changes, with closer spacing indicating steep slopes and wider spacing indicating gentle slopes. Each contour line usually has a label indicating its elevation, with the typical height between lines being 5 meters—sometimes 10 meters for more mountainous regions. By closely examining these lines, hikers can gain valuable insights into the landscape's topography and plan a route before embarking on their journey.

Contour lines always remain the same, even when woods get cut down or structures are torn down, making them the most reliable features on the map for finding your way. Orient yourself and the map until what you see in front of you matches the contour lines on the map. Next, you can look for natural features, like rivers, lakes, and forests, and for man-made structures to see if they match up.

Grid Coordinates

Grid coordinates are a system that allows precise location identification. Each system is specific to only the map you are using. The map is divided into a grid pattern formed by intersecting vertical lines (eastings) and horizontal lines (northings). Each line represents a specific numerical value. To determine a grid coordinate identify the easting line on the bottom of the map. Next, locate the northing line on the left of the map and move horizontally until it intersects the easting line. The grid coordinate is the intersection of the chosen easting and northing lines, pinpointing the exact location on the map. When quoting a grid coordinate, you give the eastings first, then the northings. An easy way to remember the order of description is to think about going "along the hall and up the stairs."

GPS Coordinates

Some international maps use latitude and longitude, like GPS, instead of grid coordinates. While a grid coordinate relies on a specific map grid system, a GPS coordinate is universally understood and can be used across different mapping applications and GPS devices.

A GPS coordinate consists of a horizontal line of latitude and a vertical line of longitude. Latitude measures degrees of distance north or south of the equator, ranging from 0 at the equator to 90 degrees at the north pole and negative 90 degrees at the south pole. Longitude measures degrees of distance east or west of the Prime Meridian, ranging from zero at the Prime Meridian to 180 degrees east and negative 180 degrees to the west.

Whether or not you have a GPS device with you, it's a good idea to have a backup map and compass in case it either becomes damaged or lost.

USING A COMPASS

A compass is a basic but vital tool for navigating the outdoors, allowing you to determine directions and orient yourself in relation to your surroundings. It requires no batteries and works with any map. It works based on the Earth's magnetic field and the principles of magnetism. Understanding how a compass functions and how to use it along with a topographical map will greatly enhance your navigation skills.

The basic design of a compass consists of a magnetized needle, usually red at one end, that is balanced on a pivot point. The needle aligns itself with the Earth's magnetic field, which has a magnetic north and south pole. The direction that the red end of the needle points to is called the magnetic north. That is the main thing to know about a compass. It points to the magnetic north. All other data relies on that simple fact.

Beware though, that metallic objects, magnets, and electronic devices can interfere with the compass needle, and therefore, they should be kept at a distance while working with a compass. Some locations around the world also have geographical features that interfere with compasses, for instance, the Cuillin mountain range in Scotland which are largely composed of ferromagnetic materials.

It's important to familiarize yourself with and understand the functions of the various parts of the compass. If possible, have a compass to hand while you go through this section. That will make it much easier to follow and understand.

- The baseplate is the clear plate that the compass is mounted in.
- The direction-of-travel arrow is the stationary arrow printed on the baseplate.
- The needle housing contains the bezel, magnetized needle, orienting arrow, and orienting lines.
- The rotating bezel or azimuth ring is the outer ring around the needle housing and has 360-degree markings on it.
- The orienting arrow is the printed outline in the shape of the magnetized end of the needle. It moves when you adjust the declination of the compass.
- The orienting lines rotate along with the bezel. When you align the orienting lines with the north-south lines on the map, the orienting arrow will point north.

- The index line is the point on the base plate that is directly in line with the direction-of-travel arrow and next to the bezel. It is used to mark the bearing you set when you rotate the bezel.

When using a compass in combination with a topographical map, follow these steps to navigate effectively:

1. Adjust the declination on the compass. This is very important, as magnetic north and true north differ by a few degrees. You can find the declination value for the region on your topographical map, but be aware that the value also changes over time. Make sure your map is current, or consult the National Oceanic and Atmospheric Administration (NOAA) website for up-to-date values. The exact way to adjust for declination is different for every make and model of compass. Consult the information that came with the compass or the manufacturer's website.

2. Place the compass on the map, aligning the direction-of-travel arrow with the top of the map.

3. Rotate the bezel until the N aligns with the direction-of-travel arrow.

4. Align the straight edge of the baseplate to the left or right side of the map.

5. Hold the compass level and steady, and rotate your body until the magnetic needle aligns with the orienting arrow.

6. Now, you can use topographical map features, such as contour lines, to identify landmarks, valleys, ridges, or other recognizable terrain features. Compare them to what you see in the actual landscape to confirm your location on the map.

Taking Bearings

A bearing is a more precise way of saying which direction you are traveling in. Your bearing is relative to your location and your destination.

Here is how you take a bearing:

1. Align the straight edge of the baseplate with where you are and where you want to go. The direction-of-travel arrow should point in the same general direction.

2. Rotate the bezel to align the orienting lines to the north-south grid lines on the map. Make sure N is pointing north on the map.

3. Read the degree marking at the index line. This is your current bearing.

4. Pick up your compass, and point the direction-of-travel arrow away from you.

5. Rotate your body until the magnetic needle aligns with the orienting arrow. You've now aligned the direction-of-travel arrow with your bearing, and you can follow it to your destination.

You can also take bearings by sight to determine where you are on a trail or even where you are on the map when you don't have a trail as a guide.

1. Find a landmark that you can identify on both the map and in front of you.
2. Hold the compass level, and point the direction-of-travel arrow at the landmark.
3. Rotate the bezel until the magnetic needle aligns with the orienting arrow.
4. Place the compass on the map, aligning the top corner of the straight edge of the base plate with the landmark.
5. Rotate the whole baseplate to align the orienting lines to the north-south grid lines on the map, making sure that the direction-of-travel arrow is still pointing at the landmark. The N on the bezel should now point north on the map.
6. Draw a line along the straight edge. Your location on the trail will be where the line from the landmark intersects your trail.

To locate where you are on the map with some level of accuracy, you can repeat the above steps with two more landmarks. Make sure those landmarks are at least 60 degrees away from the first landmark. If done correctly, the three lines will either intersect and pinpoint your location or, more likely, make a small triangle around or near you. If your lines end up making a large triangle instead, one or more of your bearings is incorrect and you should start again.

Use your compass and topographical map together in various environments and terrains to refine your navigation skills. As you gain experience, you'll become more proficient at interpreting map features and taking accurate bearings.

PLANNING YOUR ROUTE

It's important to gather as much information as you can about your chosen trail and the surrounding region to ensure a safe and enjoyable experience. Familiarize yourself with the route before setting out. Maps, guidebooks, and online sources such as forums, blogs, and hiking platforms such as AllTrails, Gaia GPS, MapMyHike, and Wikiloc are valuable resources for trail information and user reviews. They are also a great way to discover new trails.

GPS tracks available on the abovementioned platforms offer detailed information about the trail, including ascent, descent, distance, and waypoints. They can be downloaded for handheld GPS devices, GPS watches, or smartphones equipped with GPS capabilities. This technology provides real-time positioning and navigation assistance, allowing hikers to stay on track and monitor their progress along the trail.

While electronic devices are convenient, it is still recommended to carry a printed map and a compass, especially for longer or less-marked trails. Electronic devices can break or may be unreliable due to battery drain, signal loss, or technical glitches. Printed maps and compasses offer a reliable backup and can be easily referenced without the need for batteries or connectivity.

Printed maps can be purchased online or obtained from local tourist offices. Look for topographic maps that provide detailed information about the trail, including elevation contours, landmarks, water sources, and potential hazards. These maps offer a broader perspective of the area and are invaluable for navigation, particularly in remote or less-traveled regions.

Factors to Consider When Planning Your Route

Check your chosen route for any navigational challenges, such as unmarked sections or confusing intersections. Research trip reports or connect with experienced hikers who have previously completed the trail to gain valuable insights and recommendations. Research and evaluate the necessary safety precautions for the specific trail you plan to hike.

Consider factors such as potential wildlife encounters, vegetation, ground cover, stream crossings, steep sections, or exposure to hazardous conditions. Learn about any necessary equipment—such as bear canisters, gaiters, crampons, or ice axes—that may be required for certain sections or during specific seasons. Ensure you have the appropriate knowledge, skills, and gear to handle the challenges of the trail safely.

Check if there are natural water sources available where you can refill your bottles. You might be able to save energy by not carrying as much water along. Also, remember that streams may be dry during the season you plan on hiking.

When estimating the time needed to complete the trail, consider the distance, total ascent, terrain, potential obstacles, and your physical fitness level. GPS tracks often provide an estimated duration based on average hiking speeds. However, it is necessary to adjust this estimate based on your own capabilities. Choose a trail that matches your physical capabilities and experience. Start with shorter and less challenging hikes if you're a beginner, gradually increasing the difficulty as your fitness and skills improve. If hiking with others, it is recommended to base the required time on the least fit person in the group to ensure everyone can hike comfortably and avoid rushing or exhausting themselves. Also, consider factors such as rest breaks and any planned stops for photography, lunch, or sightseeing. Weather conditions and trail congestion can also affect your pace. It is better to allocate more time than necessary and allow for flexibility in your schedule to accommodate any unforeseen circumstances.

Consider any specific requirements or permits associated with the trail. Some trails may have entry fees, limited access, or require advance reservations. Research the regulations and plan accordingly to ensure compliance and avoid any disappointment or inconvenience on the day of your hike.

Consider the season and elevation of the trail when planning your hike. Different seasons bring varied weather conditions which can significantly affect trail conditions and safety. Understand the trail's exposure to elements, potential temperature changes, and any specific seasonal challenges such as snow in winter, mud in early spring, the rainy season, and daytime temperatures. The amount of daylight available also changes with the season, you might need a headlamp or flashlight to hike in the dark. Higher elevations may experience colder temperatures and stronger winds, so dress and prepare accordingly.

WHAT TO DO IF YOU GET LOST

Nobody plans on getting lost; nevertheless, it still happens to many hikers. As a precaution, you could do the following:

- Stay aware of your surroundings. Look out for landmarks while you're hiking that you can easily identify and follow in case you lose your direction.
- If you've been taking pictures, they may help you remember your way or you could scan them for familiar landmarks.
- You can make temporary markers along your trail to help you find your way back using rocks, sticks, or trail-marking ribbons, but make sure to take them down when you pass by them again.

Preparedness is the key to not getting lost in the first place, but what if, despite your best efforts you still end up disoriented? The U.S. Forest Service recommends you remember STOP:

- **Stop**: If you think you might be lost, stop immediately and stay put. Stay calm, and don't go any further just yet.
- **Think**: Try to remember your way back. Go over the path you took in your mind. Have a look at any photos you may have taken to see if they jog your mcmory.
- **Observe**: Have a look around to see if you recognize any landmarks around you. Use your compass to reorient yourself. Check your map to see if you can determine your location. If you are still on a trail, stay on it. As a last resort only, follow a stream or

drainage pipe downhill. You are bound to find a trail or a road on your way.

- **Plan**: Come up with a plan based on your observations. If you are still unsure or you are tired, it's best to stay put for a while, maybe even until morning. Once you are refreshed, you'll be able to think more clearly and make rational decisions.

Once you've thought it through, your possible plans of action are:

- Retrace your steps to find your way along or to the path again. If the weather is hot, avoid hiking between 10 a.m. and 4 p.m. to prevent dehydration and heatstroke. Also, avoid eating while hiking as your body won't be able to digest the food properly. Find some shade, and take a break for at least 30 minutes—longer if you are still feeling tired before carrying on.
- Check your phone for coverage, and call for help if possible.
- Stay where you are.

If you would rather stay and wait for potential rescuers, you will need to employ some vital survival skills:

- If you don't have a shelter, you'll need to create an emergency lean-to shelter using a tarp or branches.

There's no telling how long you'll be there, so prepare yourself to spend at least one night.

- Temperature extremes can be very dangerous. Create a small, contained fire to keep yourself warm. Your shelter will also provide shade during hot days.
- Stay hydrated. Seek out a source of water, and boil it before drinking. The last thing you want to do is get sick as well. A heat-safe plastic container filled with water will not burn or melt in a fire. Improvise a tripod and hang the container high above the fire.
- Hang brightly colored clothing or gear in the area around you so that your location will be more visible from above.
- During daylight hours, create a rescue signal by using rocks to spell SOS in a clearing, flashing light at potential rescuers using a reflective surface, using a whistle to make noise, or making a controlled but smoky fire and attempting some smoke signals.
- Try to conserve energy, and rest whenever you are tired.
- If you are wounded, wash your wounds thoroughly to avoid infection.

SUMMARY

- Learning how to use a topographical map and compass are essential skills for any hiker.

- All maps have a legend to help you identify and understand the map features.
- Learning how grid and GPS coordinates work makes it easy for you and others to know where the location that you are referencing is.
- Planning your route is necessary for a successful hike.
- In the event that you become lost during a hike, remember to STOP: stop, think, observe, and plan.
- Learning survival skills can save your life in the event that you get lost in the wild.

Now that you've learned the art of navigation including using a map and compass, planning your route, and what to do in the event that you get lost, you should begin noticing the positions of landmarks all around you and how they relate to where you are in the world. In the next chapter, we'll be looking at the fitness aspect of planning your hike so that you will be physically ready to take on the challenges of the trail.

4

YOUR BODY AND HIKING

Your body is designed for movement and hiking is one of the best ways to honor that design.

— UNKNOWN

ASSESSING YOUR FITNESS LEVEL

I t can be hard to know if you are fit enough to go hiking without experiencing the trail firsthand. The best way to be certain is to assess your fitness level regularly by doing some type of benchmark test. Attempt such a test on a monthly basis to see if your training is paying off.

The easiest way is to attempt a simple step test. This hiking fitness assessment requires no equipment or complicated calculations and allows you to gauge your endurance and lower body strength, giving you an indication of your current hiking fitness level.

How to Conduct a Simple Step Test

1. Find a step or a suitable, sturdy object that you can step up and down on. A step that falls between half and three-quarters the height of your shin is an appropriate level of challenge for the test.
2. Set a timer for 10–30 minutes. The duration of the test is based on your current fitness level. If you are a beginner or you've not trained a lot yet, start with a shorter time, and increase the duration once you've had more experience or if you find the test is too easy for you.
3. Complete as many steps as possible within the timeframe. Begin stepping up and down on the chosen step, maintaining a steady pace throughout the test and alternating which leg steps up first. Count the number of steps completed within the time limit.
4. Record your results. Keep track of the number of steps you accomplished during the test as it will serve as your baseline measurement.
5. Although optional, adding a weighted pack while doing the step test can simulate hiking with a loaded

backpack. This enhances the test's accuracy and prepares you for the demands of hiking with a load.

Repeating the assessment every four to six weeks allows you to monitor your progress over time. Aim to conduct the test under similar conditions, using the same step height, duration, and pack weight each time.

As you progress in your training, focus on increasing the number of steps completed during the designated time frame. This improvement indicates enhanced cardiovascular endurance and lower body strength. By comparing your results from each test, you can assess your training's effectiveness, identify areas for improvement, and if necessary, adjust your training program accordingly.

Remember, the step test serves only as a general assessment of your hiking fitness and should be combined with other exercises and activities to achieve overall fitness. Incorporate cardio workouts, strength training, and hiking-specific exercises into your routine to optimize your hiking performance. Always listen to your body, progress gradually, and consult with a healthcare professional before starting a new exercise program, especially if you have any pre-existing health conditions.

The YMCA Three-Minute Step Test

Testing your cardiovascular fitness is just as essential as testing your endurance. The simplest way to do this is to complete the YMCA three-minute step test. You will require a step that is 12 inches tall, a stopwatch, and a metronome. A cell phone and app will do for the latter two requirements.

Before starting, get to know the pace of the metronome when set to 96 beats per minute (bpm). You'll need to complete one step up or down with both feet every time the metronome ticks, in other words: right up, left up, tick, right down, left down, tick. Focus on your posture while you do this, and keep your back straight.

1. Set a timer for three minutes, and set the metronome to 96 bpm.
2. After three minutes, take your pulse immediately. Do this by finding the spot on your wrist at the base of your thumb using your fore and middle fingers. Count how many times your heart beats in 60 seconds, and write it down, along with the date, for future reference.
3. Refer to the chart below for your result.

Heart Rates After Completing the YMCA Three-Minute Step Test (in Beats Per Minute)

Age	18–25		26–35		36–45		46–55		46–65		65+	
Gender	Male	Female	Male	Female	Male	Female	Male	Female	Male	Female	Male	Female
Excellent	50–76	52–81	51–76	58–80	49–76	51–84	56–82	63–91	60–77	60–92	59–81	70–92
Good	79–84	85–93	79–85	85–92	80–88	89–96	87–93	95–101	86–94	97–103	87–92	96–101
Above Average	83–93	96–102	88–94	95–101	92–88	100–104	95–101	104–110	97–100	106–111	94–102	104–111
Average	95–100	104–110	96–102	104–110	100–105	107–112	103–111	113–118	103–109	113–118	104–110	116–121
Below Average	102–107	113–120	104–110	113–119	108–113	115–120	113–119	120–124	111–117	119–127	114–118	123–126
Poor	111–119	122–131	114–121	122–129	116–124	124–132	121–126	126–132	119–128	129–135	121–126	128–133
Very Poor	124–157	135–169	126–191	134–171	130–163	137–169	131–159	137–169	131–154	141–174	130–151	135–155

To improve your cardiovascular efficiency, you will need to incorporate cardio workouts—such as running, cycling, aerobics, stair climbing, etc.—into your workout plan. As a variation on the three-minute step test, you can do the following workout:

1. Set a metronome to 96 bpm.
2. Do 15 step-ups, then 15 more with the other leg leading.
3. Rest until your heart rate has recovered.
4. Repeat steps one and two twice more.

Optionally, do this exercise with a weighted backpack or while holding two 10-pound weights.

FOOD

Hiking is physically demanding and consumes a large amount of energy. The combination of walking, climbing, and navigating uneven terrains requires the engagement of various muscle groups and the cardiovascular system.

The body relies on ingested carbohydrates and ingested and stored fats to fuel the muscles during prolonged hikes. To meet our bodies' energy demands, we hikers need to consume an adequate amount of calories and stay properly hydrated. Planning and packing nutritious snacks, meals, and sufficient water are essential for maintaining energy levels and maximizing hiking performance.

What to Pack

If you're planning on spending the whole day hiking, you might not want to go through a lot of hassle when preparing dinner once you set up camp, so more snacks and simpler meals might be a better choice for you.

Most of the time you'll be able to bring along a dehydrated or compact version of the foods you like. Comfort foods keep your spirits high and are a powerful motivator when hiking a tough trail. Good food will taste even better at the end of a long day. These days there are loads of companies making ready-to-eat camping foods such as mushroom risotto, Indian korma, macaroni and cheese, and many other lightweight dehydrated foods, so there are loads of tasty options to choose from.

How Much to Pack

There are a few considerations when deciding how much food to pack. A more intense hike means more energy is required. The length of the trail, the number of days out, terrain, walking pace, your weight, the weight of your pack, and the elevation gained are a few of the factors that will influence how intense your hike will be.

On a hike of average intensity, 1½ to 2½ pounds of food, or 2,500 to 4,500 calories, should be enough per person per day. It's a good idea to always take an extra day's worth of food along in the event of a delay or other unforeseen circumstances.

Dehydrated Meals

Dehydrated meals are a popular food option for hikers and outdoor enthusiasts due to their lightweight nature, convenience, and long shelf lives. These meals undergo a dehydration process that removes most of their water content, reducing their weight significantly while preserving their nutritional value.

Weight is a critical consideration when planning a hiking trip, especially for multiday or long-distance hikes. Dehydrated meals are incredibly lightweight compared to traditional food options. By removing the moisture, meals become compact and lightweight, allowing you to carry a substantial amount of food without adding excessive weight to your backpack. They are also designed to be quick and easy to prepare, requiring minimal cooking equipment and preparation time. Most meals only require adding hot water directly to the package, saving you time and fuel while on the trail. This convenience is particularly valuable when hiking in remote areas or during adverse weather conditions when setting up a full cooking setup may be impractical.

Dehydrated meals are carefully crafted to provide a balance of essential nutrients required for sustained energy during outdoor activities. These meals are often designed to be high in carbohydrates, moderate in protein, and contain the necessary fats and fiber. They typically include a variety of ingredients such as grains, legumes, vegetables, and meats, providing a well-rounded and satisfying meal. Many dehydrated meals also cater to specific dietary preferences or restrictions, offering vegetarian, vegan, and gluten-free options. You can also select from an array of flavors, portion sizes, and spice levels to suit your taste and nutritional needs.

Dehydrated food has an extended shelf life, making it suitable for long trips or emergency situations. Because the dehydration process removes moisture, it inhibits the growth of bacteria and other microorganisms that can spoil food. This longer shelf life allows you to plan and pack meals in advance without the concern of them spoiling or needing refrigeration during your trip.

If you own a food dehydrator, you can also create your own dehydrated meals at home by dehydrating your favorite recipes. This allows you the ability to customize your dehydrated meals by adding extra spices, herbs, or ingredients to modify them according to your individual taste preferences and providing a level of control over everything that goes into your meal. Though it requires more work, it will be much cheaper to make your own dehydrated meals.

While dehydrated meals offer the benefits of convenience and reduced weight, it's important to consider a few factors when relying on them for extended periods. First, dehydrated meals may lack the same freshness and texture as freshly prepared food. Second, they may have higher sodium content to enhance flavor and act as a preservative, so it's essential to maintain proper hydration. Lastly, dehydrated meals may not provide the same sensory experience and comfort as a hot, freshly cooked meal, which can be a significant consideration for some hikers. Take some extra spices and a wide variety of flavors so that your taste buds won't get bored.

Overall, dehydrated meals are an excellent option for hiking, saving weight, ensuring proper nutrition, and providing convenience on the trail. They offer you the opportunity to enjoy a satisfying meal with minimal effort, which is especially welcome after completing a grueling day on the trail.

Lightweight and Easy Meal Options

To avoid carrying unnecessary extra weight, plan and pack lightweight and easy meal options that provide enough nutrition and satisfy your hunger. Dehydrated meals are a popular choice, but there are other snacking alternatives that offer variety and simplicity as well.

Wraps and sandwiches are versatile and portable meal options. Choose durable bread or tortillas that won't easily get squished during your hike. Fill them with a variety of ingredients such as deli meats, cheese, hummus, vegetables, and spreads. These are great for eating during your first day or two on the trail. Opt for ingredients that are less perishable and won't spoil quickly.

Trail mix and snack bars are quick and convenient options that provide energy on the go. Prepare your own trail mix by combining nuts, dried fruits, seeds, and maybe even a bit of chocolate or granola. Snack bars come in various flavors and can be packed with nutritious ingredients. Look for options with minimal packaging to reduce waste.

Prepackaged tuna or chicken pouches are lightweight and a good source of protein. They can be enjoyed on their own or mixed with mayonnaise, mustard, or other condiments for a simple and satisfying meal. Consider single-serve packets to minimize weight and waste.

Instant noodles or rice are lightweight and require minimal preparation. Look for options that can be prepared with hot water only. While not eliminating the need for a stove, they do save on fuel. Add dehydrated vegetables, canned meats, or flavor packets to enhance the taste and nutritional value.

Lightweight and durable fruits and vegetables that won't easily spoil, such as apples, oranges, carrots, and cherry tomatoes provide essential vitamins, hydration, and a refreshing boost to your meals. Be mindful of any waste and repack peels or cores to leave no trace.

Hard cheeses like cheddar or Gouda can withstand hiking conditions and provide a welcome source of protein and fat. Pair them with sturdy crackers that won't crumble easily.

Individual servings of nut butter in portable packets are a convenient and high-energy option. Enjoy them on their own, as a dip for fruit or vegetables, spread on crackers or tortillas, or mix them with other ingredients for a quick and satisfying snack.

Instant oatmeal or cereal packets are lightweight and require minimal cooking. They can be prepared by adding hot water or cold milk if you opt to take some along. Look for options with added nuts, seeds, or dried fruits for added nutrition and flavor.

Some prepackaged meals—like canned soups, stews, or chili —can be lightweight and convenient if you're not concerned about the added weight. Opt for low-sodium or healthy options whenever possible. Transfer the contents into a lightweight container or resealable bag to save space and cut down on weight.

Consider using lightweight and collapsible containers for storing your meals. These containers can be washed and reused throughout your hike, reducing waste and saving space in your backpack.

Remember to pack enough water or bring a water filtration system to stay hydrated while enjoying your meals—but make sure that there are natural water sources along the trail if you are opting to largely use filtered water. Customize your meal plan according to your preferences, dietary restrictions, and nutritional needs. Practice Leave No Trace principles by packing out any waste and disposing of it properly. With careful planning and consideration, you can enjoy delicious and nourishing meals while keeping your backpack light.

KEEPING CLEAN

Keeping clean while hiking is important for personal hygiene, comfort, and overall well-being. When you've been on the trail for a long time, the line between hiker and homeless can blur, especially from an outsider's perspective on occasions when you re-enter society.

Prepare a hygiene kit that includes items such as biodegradable soap, a toothbrush, toothpaste, toilet paper, wet wipes, hand sanitizer, a towel, and other hygiene products. Take travel-sized items along to save space in your backpack.

Changing into clean clothes helps prevent skin irritation, chafing, and the accumulation of dirt and sweat. It also provides a psychological boost, making you feel refreshed and rejuvenated. Store used clothes in a separate waterproof bag to keep them away from the clean ones and maintain organization in your backpack.

Prevent dirt, sweat, and tangles by tying your hair up or wearing a hat or bandana. This helps to keep your hair cleaner and more manageable during the hike. It also protects your scalp from the sun and minimizes the accumulation of dust and debris.

Extended hikes can lead to body odor due to sweating. Pack a small travel-sized deodorant or body spray to manage odor and keep yourself feeling fresh. Look for products that are environmentally friendly and have minimal packaging.

Drinking plenty of water is not only essential for your overall health but also helps flush out toxins from your body, keeping you feeling fresh. Proper hydration also contributes to maintaining healthy skin and preventing dehydration-related issues. Carry a sufficient amount of water, and drink regularly throughout your hike.

Carrying a lightweight, quick-drying towel or even a bandana is useful for various purposes. You can use it to dry off after cleaning yourself and to wipe away sweat during the hike. Moreover, if temperatures rise suddenly, the cloth can be soaked in water and draped or tied over key arteries at the neck and wrists to keep you cool and reduce the body's need to sweat. Look for compact towels made from microfiber materials that are absorbent and dry quickly, saving space and weight in your backpack.

Look for a campsite that offers amenities such as clean water sources, toilet facilities, and access to a shower or bathing area. This will make it easier to maintain cleanliness throughout your stay.

It's important to keep clean, even while hiking. Bathing options may be limited, especially in remote areas, but consider options such as sponge baths with a small amount of water, using biodegradable soap and a washcloth. Even without soap, you can still wash sweat off, because sweat is water soluble.

Alternatively, if you're camping near a water source, you can take a dip or swim to clean yourself, even to rinse out used clothes. Use eco-friendly products to minimize your impact on the environment. However, some national parks and other areas may have restrictions in place against bathing or entering rivers or natural water sources, so make sure to familiarize yourself with the rules.

Dry shampoo can be a handy option for refreshing your hair without access to running water.

Quick-drying and moisture-wicking fabrics for clothing can help manage sweat and odor, keeping you feeling cleaner for longer periods between washes. Have a separate set of clothes to sleep in to avoid contaminating your sleeping bag with bad smells.

For menstruation: Dispose of menstrual cup contents in a 6-inch (15 cm) deep hole, called a cat hole, and pack up used tampons or pads as animals will dig them up.

Maintain cleanliness around your campsite by keeping it free of trash and food waste. Dispose of waste properly by using designated trash receptacles or packing up your garbage. Cleaning up after yourself not only helps preserve the natural environment but also ensures a more enjoyable camping experience for yourself and others. If you're in a remote area where there is nowhere for you to dispose of trash, take it with you until you can dispose of it properly.

Brush your teeth at least twice a day to maintain oral health. Use biodegradable toothpaste and a small amount of water. Spit the toothpaste into a designated hole 200 ft away from natural water sources, or dispose of it properly to avoid contamination.

Wash your dishes, utensils, and cookware thoroughly after use. Use hot water and biodegradable soap, if available, to eliminate grease and food residue. Properly dispose of gray water 200 ft from water sources.

Remember, maintaining cleanliness while camping not only ensures personal comfort but also helps preserve the natural environment for future hikers. Respect the wilderness, and follow Leave No Trace principles by leaving the trail cleaner than when you found it.

WHAT TO DO ABOUT POO

When nature calls during your outdoor adventures, it's important to properly and hygienically dispose of poo by following Leave No Trace principles to maintain the natural beauty of outdoor spaces, protect the environment, and ensure the safety of wildlife and other hikers.

If there are no established facilities, find a secluded area at least 200 ft away from water sources, the campsite, and the trail to conduct business. Use a trowel, stick, tent peg, or rock to dig a cat hole six to eight inches deep, and fill it back in to cover it properly after use. The depth is important to ensure proper decomposition and to discourage animals from digging it up. Always practice good hygiene by washing your hands with soap and water or using hand sanitizer afterward.

Don't wait until it's an emergency to find a suitable spot. Plan ahead, and be aware of your surroundings. Identify potential locations for cat holes along your hiking route and familiarize yourself with Leave No Trace principles.

To prevent wildlife from digging up toilet paper, place used toilet paper in a sealable bag and dispose of it properly when you reach a trash receptacle.

In certain environmentally sensitive areas where packing up human waste is required, consider using commercially available poop bags designed to neutralize odors and turn liquid into a gel. These bags are specially designed to minimize the environmental impact. Alternatively, you can use a sealable bag or container for your poo. If you don't want to see the contents, consider wrapping tape around the bag or the container before your hike.

SUMMARY

- Assessing your fitness level with a simple step test or the YMCA's three-minute step test is an excellent way to establish whether you're fit enough to attempt longer, more strenuous hikes.
- Packing enough food to last the duration of the hike (plus an extra day's worth) is essential in maintaining your energy level.
- Having a large variety of your favorite lightweight food and snacks saves on weight, motivates, and keeps your spirits high.
- Dehydrated foods are lightweight, easy to prepare, and save on fuel.

- Good hygiene practices while on the trail are essential for your health and comfort as well as for those hiking with you.
- Utilizing cat holes properly is essential for covering human waste, preventing contamination of natural water sources, and preventing wildlife from coming into contact with it.

PERSONALIZED FITNESS TESTS

If you'd like to come up with your own fitness tests for hiking, there are a few things that the test must be able to do to be considered a good assessment:

- **Not just any random fitness test will do:** Speed tests—like the beep test that has you running back and forth across a distance of 10 yards at decreasing time intervals—aren't very useful for hiking, in general, unless you are a trail runner. The test needs to be relevant to hiking like the simple step test. Consider the types of obstacles you'll face on the trail, like inclines, rough terrain, or even short climbs.
- **You need to be able to measure each test in order to record it:** You won't be able to tell whether you improved over time or not unless you are able to measure your performance and can reference previous measurements.

- **Your test should be repeatable:** You'll need to be able to set up the conditions in the same way every time in order to accurately assess your progress—for instance, the same time interval, number of repetitions, weight, and distance or height.
- **Keep it simple:** Unless you have a coach or fitness trainer to assess your form and guide you through an exercise, you will need to stick to very basic exercises involving mostly your legs but also, to a lesser degree, your core and upper body.

Now that we've discussed the importance of being fit and assessing your fitness before hitting the trail, keeping your body energized, and practicing good hygiene while hiking, we can have a look at what to do when the unforeseeable happens. Despite taking every precaution, accidents that require medical attention can still happen.

If you are enjoying this book and finding it to be helpful, we would kindly like to ask you to leave a brief review on Amazon.

Reviews are not easy to come by, but they have a profound impact. Leaving a review is not just about sharing your thoughts, it's about helping your fellow hikers make informed decisions. So, we would be incredibly thankful if you would take a minute or two to leave a quick review.

Here is a link: https://www.amazon.com/review/create-review/?asin=[ASIN]

Or, Visit Amazon, find The Hiker's Companion for Beginners by Drake Evans, click on "Write a review", share your thoughts and anything you gained from the book, and hit the "Submit" button. It does not need to be long.

Thank you. We are appreciative.

5

FIRST-AID GUIDE

First aid is the immediate bridge between injury and recovery.

— UNKNOWN

GENERAL FIRST AID

Nobody plans on getting injured, especially on the trail, far from civilization. First-aid skills and preparedness are of extreme importance when venturing into the wilderness on hiking expeditions. It's essential to have at least a basic first-aid kit with you at all times when you're hiking. You can also put together a first-aid kit of your own, or add supplies to it as you go along. Regularly check product expiry dates, and replenish your supplies to keep the kit up-to-date. At the end of this chapter, you'll find a checklist of all the essential items your first-aid kit should include.

It's important to familiarize yourself with basic first-aid techniques and wilderness medicine so that you'll be ready in the event of an emergency. Take the time to educate yourself on common injuries and illnesses that can occur during hiking, such as cuts, scrapes, blisters, sprains, fractures, heat exhaustion, hypothermia, and allergic reactions. Understand the signs and symptoms associated with these conditions, and know how to provide initial care and seek appropriate medical assistance. Familiarize yourself with proper wound care, bandaging techniques, and how to respond to emergencies.

Clean and disinfect wounds like cuts, scrapes, and blisters using antiseptic wipes or solutions to prevent infection. Apply sterile dressings or bandages to cover and protect wounds. Use adhesive bandages or blister pads to treat blisters and provide relief.

Carry pain relievers and anti-inflammatory medication in your first-aid kit to manage pain and inflammation caused by minor injuries. Follow the appropriate dosage instructions, and consult with a healthcare professional if needed.

Be aware of the signs and symptoms of allergic reactions, including insect stings, plant exposure, or food allergies. Carry appropriate medications such as antihistamines or epinephrine (if prescribed) to manage severe allergic reactions. Be mindful of any known allergies within your hiking group, and be careful when sharing food that may contain allergens.

Cardiopulmonary resuscitation (CPR) can be a life-saving intervention during emergencies. Stay updated on CPR techniques, and know how to perform them if necessary. Consider taking a wilderness first aid or wilderness first responder course for more comprehensive training on emergency response in remote environments.

Remember, prevention is always better than treatment. Being well-prepared and knowledgeable in first aid can contribute to a safer hike and may even save a life.

DEALING WITH FOOT PROBLEMS

Most injuries and pain you will encounter on the trail will involve your feet. They will likely need to carry you for a few more miles, so taking care of your feet is very important. There are plenty of boots, socks, and insoles on the market designed with maximum comfort in mind, but try as you might, you can never fully eliminate foot problems when hiking.

As always, prevention is better than a cure. Condition and treat your feet before and during your hike to ensure they will carry you where you want to be with as few problems as possible.

- For one to two weeks before you hit the trail, soak your feet for 20 minutes every night in an Epsom salt solution. Afterward, moisturize them thoroughly using an anti-friction foot cream, and wear lightweight socks to bed.
- Check your socks and shoes for any debris like sticks and rocks. Even a small pebble can rub against your foot while you walk causing abrasions, blisters, and possibly even damage to your insoles or socks. Stop and remove debris as soon as you feel it to prevent further damage. Wearing gaiters is an effective way of keeping the trail from getting into your shoes.
- As you hike, pay attention to any sensations of hot spots on your feet, which may indicate areas of friction and potential blisters. It's best to stop and address the issue immediately to prevent it from getting worse. Apply moleskin, blister tape, or an antifriction moisturizer to the affected area to reduce further irritation. If you've already developed a blister, treat it correctly to avoid infection and further discomfort: Clean the area with antiseptic wipes, puncture the blister with a sterilized needle, and drain the fluid gently. Apply an antibiotic

ointment, and cover the blister with a sterile bandage or moleskin.

- Regularly schedule short breaks during your hike to rest and check on your feet. Remove your shoes and socks to let your feet breathe, and assess them for any developing issues like blisters or redness. Air circulation helps to dry out moisture and prevent the development of blisters and fungal infections. Take the opportunity to stretch your feet and calf muscles to relieve tension, promote blood circulation, and prevent inflammation.

- Elevate your legs and feet. Raising your feet above heart level during breaks or at the end of the day can help reduce swelling and promote better blood circulation, which helps you recover faster and minimizes foot fatigue. Including compression socks in your sleepwear can also aid in keeping blood pressure and footstep resilience consistent across long multiday hikes.

- After the day's hike, rinse your feet with cool water to remove dirt, sweat, and any irritants that may have accumulated. Treat your feet to a refreshing soak in cold water if possible. The cold water helps reduce swelling, ease soreness, and revitalize your feet, providing soothing relief after a strenuous hike. After soaking them, dry your feet thoroughly, paying special attention to the spaces between your toes, as excessive moisture can contribute to blister formation and may aggravate conditions like athlete's foot or psoriasis.

- Keep your feet and shoes dry. Wet feet—whether from sweat or a water source—cause unnecessary friction on your skin. Stop to put on dry socks once you're sure they won't get wet again, and dry your shoes as much as possible. Taking out the insoles will help your shoes dry faster. Wear moisture-wicking socks made from materials like merino wool or synthetic blends. These socks help keep your feet dry by wicking away sweat, reducing the likelihood of blisters, fungal infections, and potentially serious conditions like trench foot.

- Wearing appropriate footwear is key to foot care while hiking. Invest in sturdy, well-fitting hiking boots or shoes that provide enough support and protection. Make sure they have enough toe room to prevent toenail injuries and sufficient ankle support to reduce the risk of sprains. Consider using specialized insoles or orthotics in your hiking shoes to provide extra support, cushioning, and stability. These insoles can improve foot alignment, reduce pressure points, and absorb shock during hikes, enhancing overall comfort and reducing the risk of foot fatigue. Customized insoles can address specific foot issues, such as overpronation or high arches. Incorrectly sized insoles may take up too much space in your shoes. This is unlikely to be the case with stock insoles. If you're using third-party insoles you haven't tried before or have limited experience with, take your shoes' stock insoles with you and swap them out in case your feet become sore.

- Rinse your hiking socks regularly during multiday hikes to remove dirt, sweat, and bacteria. Rinse them in a stream or with a water bottle and hang them to dry on the outside of your backpack while walking. Some safety pins will come in handy for this. Carrying multiple pairs of socks allows you to rotate them daily, giving each pair time to dry thoroughly and preventing excessive moisture buildup.

- At the end of the day, give your feet some TLC by gently massaging them. This helps increase blood flow, relieves pain, reduces muscle tension, and alleviates foot fatigue. Consider using a small massage ball or your hands to knead your toes and the arches and soles of your feet. You can also apply a soothing foot cream or lotion to moisturize and nourish your skin.

Common Foot Problems

- Blisters form on the skin due to friction, pressure, or rubbing against footwear. Hiking long distances or wearing ill-fitting shoes can lead to blisters, which can be painful and impede your hiking progress. If you have known trouble spots or areas prone to friction and blisters, such as heels and big toes, consider pretaping them before starting your hike. Use adhesive sports tape, moleskin, or specialized blister prevention tape to provide an extra layer of protection against friction and rubbing. Use an antifriction cream or consider foot powder to reduce moisture, especially on hot and humid days. These proactive measures can help minimize the risk of developing blisters during long hikes.

- Bunions are bony protrusions that form at the base of the big toe, causing the toe to angle inward. Hiking in narrow or ill-fitting footwear can worsen bunion pain and inflammation due to friction and pressure. If you have bunions, you should opt for hiking shoes with a wide toe box to accommodate the bunion and reduce discomfort. Using padding and wearing moisture-wicking socks can help prevent friction and minimize bunion-related pain while hiking.

- Plantar fasciitis is inflammation and pain of the thick band of tissue that connects the heel bone to the toes, called the plantar fascia. Overuse, repetitive strain, and inadequate foot support can contribute to this condition. Hikers with plantar fasciitis often experience stabbing pain in the heel, particularly in the morning or after prolonged periods of rest. Proper footwear with arch support and cushioning, stretching exercises, and rest can help manage plantar fasciitis.

- Heel spurs are bony outgrowths that form on the underside of the heel bone. They can develop alongside plantar fasciitis or due to excessive strain on the foot ligaments. Heel spurs can cause sharp pain in the heel area, especially when walking or hiking. Managing heel spurs involves addressing the underlying cause, providing proper foot support, and using cushioned insoles or heel pads to alleviate pressure on the affected area.

- Sprains occur quite often while hiking, especially on loose or uneven terrain. As soon as you feel the sprain, stop and find a comfortable spot to rest and assess the injury. Soak the injured foot in cold water or apply a first-aid instant cold compress for 15–20 minutes, and wrap it with a compression bandage for added support and limit swelling. Elevating the injured foot also reduces the swelling. Take medication to relieve some of the pain and discomfort. Avoid putting weight on the sprained foot, move carefully, and lean on your trekking poles or a sturdy stick. Once you return to camp or reach safety, rest the foot and assess its condition. If the pain persists or worsens, consult a healthcare professional.

- Hikers often face toenail issues, such as bruising, blackened toenails, or ingrown nails. These problems can arise from repetitive impact with the front of the shoe or pressure on the toes, especially during steep descents. Toenail issues can be mitigated by trimming toenails properly and wearing proper-fitting footwear with enough room for toe movement. Trim your toenails straight across and avoid cutting them too short as this can cause ingrown nails. Regularly check and maintain your toenails before heading out on a hike.

- Trench foot, also known as immersion foot, is a painful and serious condition that occurs when feet are exposed to prolonged wet and cold conditions. This can happen during hiking in wet and rainy weather or while crossing bodies of water. It is characterized by redness, swelling, thick sections of peeling and scaling skin, and an awful smell. Trench foot can lead to ulcers, infections, tissue damage, and in the worst cases, amputation and death. To prevent trench foot, ensure your feet stay dry by wearing waterproof footwear and changing into dry socks regularly. Washing your feet with warm soapy water and wiping them down with alcohol swabs are essential measures to avoid this condition.

SUMMARY

- Familiarize yourself with basic first-aid techniques and wilderness medicine, so you'll be ready in the event of an emergency.
- Always carry a basic first-aid kit while doing any kind of hiking, and keep it well-stocked.
- Carry pain relievers and anti-inflammatory medication to manage pain and inflammation caused by minor injuries.
- Stay updated on basic CPR techniques and know how to perform them if necessary.
- Wear sturdy, well-fitting hiking footwear that provides ankle support and protection.
- Prevent foot problems by taking the proper precautions.
- Stop and address foot problems immediately to prevent them from getting worse.

FIRST-AID KIT CHECKLIST

Essential Items

- antiseptic cleansing wipes
- antibacterial ointment
- an assortment of bandages
- wound-closure strips, butterfly bandages
- gauze pads of different sizes

- medical adhesive tape
- blister dressing
- pain-relief medication, including anti-inflammatories such as aspirin
- insect sting treatment
- tick remover
- rash and itch relief wipes or ointment
- antihistamines
- EpiPen (if necessary)
- sterile non-stick pads
- fine point tweezers
- safety pins
- blunt-tip scissors
- first-aid booklet, cards, or instructions
- emergency blanket
- cold packs

Additional Items to Consider

- finger splint
- structural aluminum malleable (SAM) splint
- rolled gauze
- cotton swabs
- elastic wrap
- hemostatic gauze
- liquid bandage
- triangular bandage
- antidiarrheal pills

- medication for giardiasis
- broad-spectrum antibiotics
- rehydration salts
- eye drops
- hand sanitizer
- multitool (including pliers)
- CPR mask
- surgical gloves (preferably neoprene)
- small mirror
- menstrual hygiene products

Now, assemble a first-aid kit of your own, or purchase a first-aid kit that caters specifically to hikers and outdoor use. As you gain more experience and knowledge about the types of injuries you may sustain while hiking, you can add their treatment options to your first-aid kit so that you'll always be prepared.

Now that we have learned the importance of being knowledgeable about wilderness medicine and that you should always carry a first-aid kit along to deal with injuries, we will delve into keeping safe during weather extremes, preventing bad wildlife encounters, and how to deal with whatever nature throws at you.

6

ELEMENTS OF THE ELEMENTS

In nature there are no rewards or punishments, there are consequences.

— ROBERT GREEN INGERSOLL

H iking is a phenomenal way to engage with nature and enjoy all the beautiful facets of the natural world. However, the environment itself is not without its risk factors. The sun, storms, and wildlife all have the potential to pose serious dangers if under-respected. Therefore, it is vital that we each take the necessary precautions to stay safe from the elements.

The sun is not to be trifled with. Though it can be wonderfully warm on the skin on cooler days, it can be deadly in hot weather. Recognizing the symptoms of heat exhaustion and heat stroke is critical for heat illness prevention and for staying safe during hot weather.

Heat exhaustion, if left unaddressed, can progress to heat stroke, which is a life-threatening condition, especially if you are hiking solo. Remember to prioritize your safety, and if you feel any symptoms of heat exhaustion, take immediate action to cool down and seek medical attention if necessary.

Heat stroke requires immediate action. Seek medical assistance. Being vigilant about the symptoms allows for early intervention, preventing heat-related emergencies and ensuring the safety and well-being of yourself and others during hot weather activities.

PREVENTING HEAT STROKE

- Avoid direct exposure to the sun. Seek shade during the hottest part of the day, typically from midmorning to late afternoon.
- Wear lightweight and breathable fabrics that allow air circulation, cover the skin, and wick away moisture, such as moisture-wicking shirts and pants. Loose-fitting clothes have better airflow and prevent clothes from sticking to the skin, reducing discomfort and heat retention. Light-colored

clothing reflects sunlight, keeping your body cooler compared to dark colors that absorb heat.

- Wear a wide-brimmed hat and sunglasses to protect your head and eyes from direct exposure to the sun.
- Apply sunscreen with a high SPF to exposed skin to reduce the risk of sunburn.
- Take regular breaks in shaded areas to rest and rehydrate. Staying hydrated is vital to prevent heat stroke, so listen to your body and drink before you feel thirsty. Drink cool water in small sips to help regulate your body temperature. Aim to drink at least one quart of water every two hours, adjusting this based on your activity level and how much you sweat. Carry a water bottle on the outside of your backpack or, even better, a hydration pack in your backpack to have easy access to water during the hike. Remember that other factors like high altitude and intense physical activity increase fluid loss, so be attentive to your hydration needs.
- Bring high-protein snacks while outdoors in hot weather. These snacks provide a quick energy boost and help maintain hydration levels. Opt for snacks with a good balance of protein and carbohydrates, as protein aids in muscle repair and recovery. Nuts, seeds, granola bars, and trail mix are excellent choices. These snacks not only provide sustenance but also contain essential minerals like potassium and magnesium, which aid in maintaining electrolyte

balance and preventing muscle cramps. Pairing these snacks with regular water intake enhances hydration and energy levels, reducing the risk of heat exhaustion and heat stroke.

- Find a shaded spot to rest when you feel fatigued, dizzy, or excessively sweaty. Continuous physical activity in hot weather can lead to too much heat building up in your body, increasing the risk of heat exhaustion and heat stroke. Resting in shaded areas allows the body to cool down and recover, reducing the risk of overheating. It also gives you a chance to assess your physical condition and adjust your activity level accordingly.
- Wade in a nearby body of water to help lower your body temperature, or find a shaded spot and remove any excess clothing to cool down faster. Applying wet cloths to your skin can also aid in cooling.

These measures can be life-saving in preventing heat-related illnesses.

SYMPTOMS AND TREATMENT OF HEAT EXHAUSTION AND HEAT STROKE

Treating heat exhaustion is critical to prevent it from progressing to heat stroke. Recognizing the symptoms is an important skill. Heat exhaustion can sneak up on you. Tiredness or weakness, dizziness, pale, moist skin, feeling faint, nausea, vomiting, cramps or a headache are all symptoms. They can be present in varying degrees and not all at once.

If you or someone in your group is showing signs of heat exhaustion, move them to a shaded and cool area immediately. Encourage them to rest and lie down, elevating their legs if possible. Give them water with electrolytes to sip slowly and a fatty or sugary or salty snack to eat. Avoid giving them ice-cold water as it may shock their system. Help cool them down by applying wet cloths to their skin or fanning them. If their condition worsens or does not improve, seek medical attention immediately. Prompt and appropriate treatment can help prevent heat stroke.

Heat stroke is a severe emergency that requires immediate medical assistance. If someone exhibits symptoms—a flushed face, high temperature, confusion, hallucinations, dry skin, weak and rapid pulse, seizures, or unconsciousness —it is essential to act swiftly. Call 911 if you have reception, or send someone to alert authorities while you stay with the person. While waiting for help to arrive, move the person to a shaded and cool area or, better yet, into cold water. Attempt to lower their body temperature by removing excess clothing, applying cool, damp cloths to their skin, and continuously pouring water on their head and upper body. Avoid giving them fluids to drink as they may not be able to swallow safely. Quick and appropriate treatment can be life-saving, so never hesitate to seek professional medical help for someone experiencing heat stroke.

RAIN AND STORMS

Chances are good that the rain will catch you at one point or another while you are on a hike. While possibly being an uncomfortable experience, rain itself doesn't pose an immediate threat. Here are a few tips to make the best of a rainy day on the trail:

- Keep your gear and belongings dry by using waterproof covers for your backpack and any electronic devices you may carry. Pack important items in resealable plastic bags to provide an extra layer of protection.
- Wet and slippery surfaces can increase the risk of slips and falls. Slow down your pace, take smaller steps, and use trekking poles for added stability on slippery terrain.
- Rainy weather can lead to a drop in temperature, so layer up with moisture-wicking base layers, a warm, insulating mid-layer to stay comfortable, and a waterproof and breathable rain jacket and pants to keep you dry. Consider carrying an extra set of dry clothes to change into if needed.
- Heavy rain can lead to swollen streams and rivers. Exercise caution when crossing waterways, and if in doubt, seek an alternative route or wait for the water to subside.

Lightning Safety

Mother Nature sometimes unleashes her raw power in the form of thunderstorms, with lightning as a force to be reckoned with. When you venture into the great outdoors, understanding lightning safety is paramount. Be prepared, stay informed, and use your best judgment to avoid high-risk areas during thunderstorms. By prioritizing safety and respecting the power of lightning, you can continue to enjoy your hiking adventures while minimizing potential hazards.

Lightning is a captivating but deadly phenomenon. A typical lightning bolt can reach temperatures of up to 50,000 °F — hotter than the surface of the sun—and can travel at speeds of up to 130,000 miles per hour. Its incredible force and immense energy can be destructive, causing wildfires and power outages, and most importantly, posing a significant threat to hikers caught outdoors during a thunderstorm.

One of the fundamental pillars of lightning safety while hiking is proper planning and awareness. Before heading out, check the weather forecast to gauge the possibility of thunderstorms. Keep in mind that thunderstorms can develop quickly, even if the forecast indicates clear skies at the start of your hike. Consider the following to keep safe:

- If thunderstorms are likely, consider postponing your hike or choosing lower altitude or shorter trails.

- While you're hiking, the key to staying safe is to avoid high-risk areas: Open fields, mountaintops, secluded trees, and ridges are particularly hazardous during thunderstorms, as they increase the chances of being struck by lightning due to their exposure and elevated positions.

- Seek lower ground, and take shelter in valleys or depressions, but avoid areas prone to flooding. Remember that rock overhangs may not provide sufficient protection against lightning.

- Lightning will create an electric field up to 100 ft away in all directions from where it strikes, which is dangerous as the current in the ground can still pass through you. When you are sheltering from a thunderstorm in a man-made structure or a cave, don't touch or lean against the walls as lightning always follows the path of least electrical resistance, meaning, it will pass through the walls and strike you indirectly. Stash your gear, especially trekking poles away from you. Stay away from the entrance, crouch low with your feet together, make as little contact with the ground as possible, avoid contact with the walls, and the current will pass below you harmlessly.

- Stay away from tall trees, and avoid taking refuge under lone trees, as they are more likely to attract lightning strikes. Instead, look for areas with dense stands of shorter trees and keep a safe distance from any standing water, which can also conduct electricity.

- If you're camping during a thunderstorm, avoid staying in a tent with metal poles. Opt for a low-lying area, and use your sleeping pad to insulate yourself from the ground.

- The 30-30 rule is a simple and effective guideline to estimate the distance of a thunderstorm: The time between the flash of lightning and hearing the sound can be counted to establish your distance away from the storm. If the time interval is 30 seconds or less, the thunderstorm is within six miles, and it's time to take immediate precautions. Wait at least 30 minutes after the last thunderclap before resuming your hike as lightning can strike even after the storm has passed.

- Staying informed about weather conditions is crucial when hiking. Many smartphone apps and weather radios can provide real-time updates on local weather patterns, including thunderstorms and lightning activity. Familiarize yourself with the signs of an approaching thunderstorm, such as darkening skies, distant rumbles of thunder, and increasing wind speed.

- Carry a fully stocked first-aid kit that includes materials for treating lightning-related injuries, such as burns and shock. If you're hiking in a group, have designated leaders who can make informed decisions regarding lightning safety and know how to initiate an emergency response if needed. Keep a distance of 100 ft between people until the danger has passed.

General Safety

To ensure your safety while hiking, always check the weather forecast for storms, dress appropriately, and plan your hike carefully. Be prepared for sudden weather changes and know how to respond to storms when they occur.

The great outdoors can be unpredictable, and one of the most significant natural hazards that hikers face is storms. Thunderstorms, rainstorms, and even snowstorms can quickly turn a peaceful hike into a potentially dangerous situation. Following these safety tips and using common sense, will give you peace of mind in the outdoors:

- Before heading out on your hiking journey, always check the weather forecast. Stay informed about the possibility of storms, heavy rain, or other adverse weather conditions in the area you plan to hike. If the forecast predicts severe weather, consider postponing your hike or choosing an alternative route in a safer location.
- Wearing weather-appropriate clothing is crucial for staying safe during storms: Dress in layers to regulate your body temperature and protect yourself from rain, wind, and temperature changes. A

waterproof and breathable rain jacket is a must to shield yourself from downpours, while moisture-wicking clothing can keep you comfortable even if you get sweaty during a storm.

- Be proactive, and keep an eye out for signs of an approaching storm. If you notice darkening skies, hear distant thunder, or feel a sudden drop in temperature, start seeking shelter immediately. Look for natural shelters like caves, overhangs, or dense tree canopies, but avoid taking refuge under tall trees or lone structures, as they pose a greater risk of lightning strikes.

- Avoid hiking near rivers, streams, or other bodies of water during a storm. Flash flooding can occur rapidly and without warning, turning seemingly calm waterways into dangerous torrents. Always err on the side of caution, and stay away from potential flood zones.

- If you're hiking with a group, stick together during storms, but keep some distance between others if it's a thunderstorm. Separating can increase the risk of accidents and hinder communication if someone needs help. Establish a buddy system, and ensure everyone is accounted for at all times.

- Storms can be intimidating, but it's essential to remain calm and think rationally. Avoid panic, as it can cloud your judgment and lead to rash decisions. Assess the situation carefully, and determine the best course of action based on your surroundings and the weather conditions.

- Carry a well-stocked backpack with the 10 Essentials. These items will be invaluable during emergencies and help you navigate through challenging weather conditions.

MOSQUITOS

These tiny but persistent insects can quickly turn a pleasant hike into an itchy and irritating experience. Here are a few ways you can avoid or deter them:

- Using mosquito repellent is a crucial defense against these pesky insects. Mosquitoes not only cause discomfort but can also transmit dangerous or even deadly diseases and parasites such as West Nile virus, yellow fever, and malaria. Apply a mosquito repellent containing citronella oil, DEET, picaridin, or other effective ingredients to exposed skin and clothing before hitting the trail. Reapply as needed, especially during dawn and dusk when mosquitoes are most active. Don't forget to cover all exposed areas, including your ears, neck, ankles, and wrists.
- Wearing protective clothing is a smart strategy to shield yourself from mosquito bites. Opt for lightweight, long-sleeved shirts and pants to cover as much skin as possible. Tuck pants into socks to

THE HIKERS COMPANION FOR BEGINNERS | 137

prevent mosquitoes from sneaking in. Consider wearing light colors, as mosquitoes are more attracted to dark hues. Use clothing treated with insect repellent for added protection, as mosquitos can sometimes bite through thin clothing.

- Choosing appropriate locations can play a vital role in minimizing mosquito encounters. Mosquitoes lay their eggs in stagnant water and thrive in marshy areas. Avoid hiking near ponds, marshes, or other water bodies with no current. Rather, opt for hiking trails away from these breeding grounds, such as higher elevations, open fields, or well-ventilated areas. Drier climates and windy areas are also less mosquito-prone. Research your hiking destination beforehand to identify areas with lower mosquito activity.

- Mosquitoes are drawn to thick foliage and vegetation, seeking shelter during the day and becoming more active at dusk and dawn. When choosing a campsite, opt for open areas with good air circulation and away from areas with thick undergrowth.

- Mosquito nets are lightweight and easy to carry and create a physical barrier between you and the pesky insects. When camping in areas with high mosquito activity, consider using a mosquito net around your sleeping area. This simple yet effective measure ensures a bug-free zone, providing you with a restful night's sleep and preventing potential discomfort and irritation from mosquito bites.

- Timing your hikes can be a strategic approach to avoid peak mosquito activity. Mosquitoes are most active during dawn and dusk when the weather is cooler. Plan your hikes during midmorning to early afternoon when mosquitoes are less prevalent. Also, consider hiking on windy days, as mosquitoes are less likely to fly in strong gusts.

- Staying cool can deter mosquitoes, as these insects are attracted to body heat and sweat. Wear lightweight, breathable clothing to promote air circulation and reduce sweating. Avoid overheating, and seek shaded areas to take breaks and lower your body temperature. Staying cool not only keeps mosquitoes at bay but also helps you maintain energy and focus on your hike.

- Avoid scented products like perfumes, colognes, scented lotions, or heavily scented soaps, as they can attract mosquitoes. Also be cautious with strong-smelling food and beverages, as they too may draw mosquitoes closer.

Mosquitoes aren't the only biting insects around. Don't forget to regularly check for ticks as they can transmit diseases, such as anaplasmosis, babesiosis, ehrlichiosis, Lyme disease, Powassan, rabbit fever, and the deadly Rocky Mountain Spotted Fever. After spending time outdoors, thoroughly inspect your body, clothing, and gear for ticks. Pay special attention to warm areas like armpits, groin, behind the ears, and on your scalp. If you find a tick, remove it promptly with a tick-removal tool or fine-tipped tweezers, grasping it as close to the skin's surface as possible. Pull upward with steady, even pressure to avoid leaving mouthparts behind, and place it in a sealed container for identification.

DARKNESS

Embarking on a hiking adventure under the cover of darkness can be an exhilarating and rewarding experience, adding thrill and mystery to the journey. As the sun sets, the landscape transforms, revealing a whole new world of sights and sounds. Hiking in the dark offers a chance to observe nocturnal creatures, see breathtaking nocturnal views including the unpolluted night sky, and embrace the serenity of the night. However, navigating the trails after sundown demands a heightened sense of awareness and careful preparation. In this section, we'll explore the essentials of hiking in the dark, from safety tips and gear considerations to embracing the unique challenges and wonders of the nocturnal wilderness:

- Unless you have a bright moon illuminating the trail and surrounding terrain enough to hike safely, a reliable headlamp or flashlight becomes your guiding beacon. Choose a headlamp or flashlight with sufficient brightness, adjustable settings, a red-light option, and long battery life to illuminate your path effectively. Carrying extra batteries or a backup light source is a wise precaution to prevent being left in the dark if your primary light fails. Pack spare batteries that match your headlamp or flashlight's requirements, and bring a small, reliable backup light as a failsafe.

- Be mindful of other hikers when using a headlamp or flashlight. Bright light ruins your night vision, and fully recovering it can take between 40 minutes and an hour. Opt for using red light instead as red light preserves your night vision while still allowing you to see around you.

- Trekking poles are a must-have for night hikes. They can help you maintain your balance and allow you to feel around for obstacles you may trip over.

- Do not forgo taking a map and compass. As is the case when hiking during the day, you may need navigation tools during a night hike, especially if you become lost or disoriented. You may want to familiarize yourself with objects in the night sky to help you orient yourself and guide your way in the dark.

- Familiarize yourself with the trail during daylight hours. Daylight exploration allows you to memorize landmarks, note potential obstacles and dangers, and gain a better understanding of the terrain's layout. This knowledge becomes invaluable when darkness sets in, as it helps you navigate better without relying on your headlamp or flashlight.

- Choose well-marked trails to reduce the risk of getting lost. Well-marked trails offer clear guidance, even in the absence of daylight. This minimizes the chances of straying off course and ensures you stay on the designated path.

- Stick to the trail to avoid getting lost. If nature calls and you do need to go off the trail, use a headlamp to guide your way, but if you're not too familiar with the area or the trail isn't very visible, you might want to tie one end of a rope to a nearby object and take the other end with you when you leave the trail so that you can find your way back.

- Hiking in the dark demands a more cautious and deliberate pace to ensure safety and stability. By slowing down and taking smaller steps, you maintain better balance and reduce the risk of tripping or slipping on uneven terrain. The reduced speed allows you to react promptly to obstacles and changes in the trail. It also gives your eyes more time to adjust to the darkness, enhancing your visibility and spatial awareness. Embrace the slower rhythm as it allows you to savor the nocturnal sounds and sights.

- Be cautious as uneven terrain, roots, rocks, and other obstacles will be harder to spot. Tread carefully, and stay alert to avoid potential hazards. Use your headlamp wherever necessary to scan the ground ahead, focusing on potential stumbling blocks. Taking deliberate steps and maintaining a steady pace allows you to navigate tricky sections more securely. Trust your senses, and be prepared to adjust your footing when encountering unexpected obstacles.

- Stay alert and attuned to your surroundings, listening for any unusual sounds or signs of wildlife activity. Many animals, including bears and cougars, are more active at night. The absence of visual cues heightens your other senses, which should help you detect potential dangers or wildlife encounters. Familiarize yourself with the sounds of the wilderness to differentiate harmless noises from anything of concern.

- Prioritize safety, and travel with a buddy or inform someone about your plans. Having a hiking companion provides mutual support and an extra pair of eyes in low-light conditions.

- Dress appropriately, so you'll be more visible. Wearing light-colored or reflective clothing allows your hiking companions to see you more clearly, preventing accidents or separation.

- Solo hiking in the dark can be an enlightening experience with a chance for personal growth and an opportunity to appreciate the nighttime world with minimal disturbances, but avoid hiking alone if you can help it. If circumstances demand a solo nighttime hike, exercise extra caution and remain vigilant. Prioritize familiar trails and well-lit areas, and ensure you're well-prepared with appropriate gear and navigation tools. When hiking solo in the dark, it's even more important to inform a friend or family member about your route, expected return time, and emergency contact information in case of any unforeseen circumstances.

WILDLIFE

A hike in the great outdoors brings with it the excitement of encountering fascinating wildlife. From graceful deer to majestic eagles and elusive bears, the chance to witness these creatures in their natural habitat is a thrilling experience. However, wildlife encounters also come with responsibilities and potential risks. Understanding how to interact respectfully with animals, recognizing potential hazards, and knowing how to handle encounters effectively are essential for the safety of both hikers and the wildlife itself. In this section, we will delve into the dos and don'ts of wildlife encounters while hiking in the US so that you can make informed decisions, avoid dangerous situations, and respect the incredible fauna that call these landscapes home:

- Research the local wildlife thoroughly. Understanding the potential risks and behaviors of animals in the area can help you stay safe during your adventure. Learn about common wildlife encounters, such as encounters with bears, cougars, or other potentially dangerous creatures. Familiarize yourself with their habitats, typical behavior, and how to react if you encounter them. This knowledge will allow you to take necessary precautions and avoid putting yourself or the animals in harm's way.

- Check with local park authorities, visitor centers, or online resources for updated information about recent wildlife sightings or warnings before heading out on your hike. Be aware of any recent reports of animal activity, such as bear sightings or aggressive animal behavior. If there are warnings or closures in place due to wildlife activity, it's best to heed them and choose an alternative route. Talk to other hikers or campers who have recently visited the area to gather firsthand insights.

- Making noise is an effective way to minimize the risk of surprising wildlife and initiating potentially dangerous encounters. Startling animals, such as bears or cougars, may lead to defensive behavior. Clap your hands, talk, or sing to create a consistent and audible presence as you walk. This alerts wildlife to your approach, giving them enough time to move away peacefully. Pay extra attention in areas with dense vegetation or poor visibility as these are common spots for unexpected encounters.

- Avoid hiking alone, especially in areas with known wildlife encounters. Hiking with a companion or a group increases safety and reduces the risk of unexpected animal interactions. If an encounter were to occur, having others with you can provide support and assistance in case of an emergency. Prioritize safety by staying on well-marked trails and adhering to park guidelines regarding wildlife interactions.

- Carry bear spray or other deterrents that are recommended for the specific wildlife in the area. Bear spray is a highly effective tool for deterring aggressive bears and cougars, and it can provide a valuable sense of security in cougar and bear country. Research the wildlife present in the region, and consult with local park authorities to identify the appropriate deterrents. Always have the deterrent easily accessible—ideally attached to your backpack or belt—and know how to use it effectively.

- Proper food storage is essential to minimize wildlife encounters, particularly with bears. Use bear-resistant containers or hang scented items—your food, cookware (including clean items), trash, scented hygiene products, and even the clothes you wear while cooking—in a bear bag high in a tree, away from your campsite. Also, do not cook or wash your dishes near your campsite. Bears have a keen sense of smell and are attracted to food odors, so securely storing your food will help prevent them from seeking it out. Follow the guidelines provided by park authorities, and use designated food storage areas if available. Keep your campsite clean and free of food debris, as even small traces of food can attract wildlife.

- Maintain a safe distance for both your safety and that of the animals. Never approach or attempt to feed them, as this can habituate wildlife to human presence, leading to potentially dangerous encounters. Use binoculars or a zoom camera lens to observe wildlife from afar, allowing them to behave naturally without feeling threatened. Respect their space and habitat, especially during breeding or nesting seasons when animals may be more protective or territorial. If you encounter wildlife on the trail, give them plenty of space to move away, and always yield the right of way to animals. Remember, we are visitors in their home, and it is our responsibility to ensure their safety and well-being.

The animals that may pose a danger that you are likely to encounter while hiking in the US are bears, cougars, wolves, bison, elk, moose, mountain goats, and snakes. Each of these animals has unique behaviors and responds differently to perceived threats. The following is a guide to how you should respond in the event that you come across each of these animals on your hike.

Bears

Most bears avoid human contact and will flee when they notice you, but they are unpredictable creatures, and if startled, they may respond defensively, especially if there are cubs around. Bears are most active at dawn and dusk.

If you spot a bear and it hasn't noticed you yet, you should back away slowly while keeping an eye on the bear. Never turn your back, and never run from a bear, as it may trigger an instinctual response to give chase. Get your bear spray ready, just in case it comes at you. Proceed to go around the bear, keeping a distance of 100 yards from it at all times.

It's important to make the distinction between bear species, as they typically respond in different ways to humans.

Brown or Grizzly Bears

Both names are used for the same species of bear. Those living in the coastal region of Alaska are called brown bears and are larger than inland grizzly bears due largely to differences in diet.

Grizzly bears have concave faces from their foreheads to their noses—often referred to as dish-shaped—and small, rounded ears. Their rumps are lower than their shoulders, but their most distinctive feature is a prominent shoulder hump. These bears are also quite large, reaching a height of three to five feet tall at their shoulders when standing on all fours. They have long claws with a slight curve. Their tracks can be identified by closely spaced toes all in a line with distant claw impressions.

If you encounter a grizzly bear and it has spotted you, it's important to stay calm and avert your eyes. You do not want to appear as a threat to it. Back away slowly, and talk to it in a low, calm voice. Keep backing away, and get to a distance of at least 100 yards, even if the bear backs down.

They may bluff charge you with the intention of scaring you away, but as difficult as it may be in a situation like this, keep calm and stand your ground. They will have their ears up and make a lot of noise while coming at you, but they will usually stop.

Have your bear spray ready in case it does charge at you for real. In this case, they'll come at you silently, with their heads lowered and ears pulled back. If they are within 30 ft of you, it is a good time to use your bear spray. Aim low, and spray it in short bursts as it comes toward you so that it passes through the stinging cloud of spray. If all else fails, you should play dead by lying on your stomach with your feet wide apart, hands protecting the back of your neck, and remaining calm. It may try to flip you over, but keep rolling back onto your stomach. The bear should lose interest soon enough.

Black Bears

Don't let the name fool you. Black bears can be a variety of colors, including brown, so identification by color is not reliable. These bears can be found in most regions and are the most common species.

Black bears have a straight face profile from their foreheads to their noses and have prominent, slightly pointy, oval ears. Their rumps are higher than their shoulders, and they don't have the characteristic shoulder hump and low rump of grizzly bears. These bears are smaller than grizzlies, standing two to three-and-a-half feet tall at their shoulders when they're on all fours. They have short, curved claws. Their tracks can be identified by arced, separated toes with claw impressions near the pads.

If you encounter a black bear and it has spotted you, scare it off by making a lot of noise and back away slowly. Avoid making high-pitched noises like whistling or shrieking as it might draw the bear closer. Try to appear as large as possible by raising your arms or trekking poles above your head or swinging an item of clothing overhead.

If the bear continues to approach you, use your bear spray, and if all else fails and it attacks, you'll need to get physical.

Use whatever you have around you as a weapon, or punch it in the neck, eyes, or nose until it backs off.

Cougars or Mountain Lions

Also known as pumas, these are elusive animals that mostly inhabit the western US and Canada but are sometimes found in the eastern states. They are mostly active at night, so avoid night hiking in areas where cougars have been spotted. They tend to keep their distance from humans, but if one were to approach you, stand your ground and don't run. Try to scare it by making a lot of noise, and back away slowly. Try to appear as large and threatening as possible. If it persists, you should use bear spray to deter it and fight back with whatever you have at hand.

Wolves

Wolves avoid humans in the wild. In the extremely unlikely event that they do attack, they have likely been habituated to humans, or they are responding to hikers with dogs. Do not run away, but make yourself appear larger and as threatening as possible, maintain eye contact, and slowly back away. Be aggressive or use bear spray if they don't retreat and keep acting aggressively.

Bison

Bison may not appear to be threatening, but when provoked, they can close the distance between you and them in moments. Keep a distance of 25 yards or more from them at all times, and don't try to scare them.

If a bison is aggressive, it will show it by snorting, bobbing its head, pawing, or bluff charging. Get behind a tree or boulder for safety, but don't attempt to outrun them, as they can reach speeds of up to 40 miles per hour.

Elk

Elk can attack when they feel threatened and are quite aggressive in the fall during mating season. Keep a distance of 50 yards or more from them, and give them a wide berth. If they do attack, get behind a tree or boulder for safety.

Moose

Moose usually aren't aggressive animals, but they may try to defend themselves if they feel threatened. When threatened, the hair on their backs will be raised, and they will pull their ears back. Back away slowly, but if it charges, run or get behind a tree or boulder. It shouldn't chase you far. Do not fight back, and if it manages to get to you, curl up into a ball and protect your head.

Mountain Goats

Mountain goats rarely attack and usually keep away from humans. When they do approach, it is likely that they have been habituated to humans. They may be attracted by the smell of sweat and urine and associate humans with a source of minerals. Keep a distance of 50 yards or more from them.

If they approach and seem aggressive, chase them off by making noise, or fight back with whatever you have at hand.

Snakes

Snakes are unlikely to initiate an attack unless they feel threatened. Unless you can positively identify the snake as nonvenomous, treat it as potentially dangerous. Keep a safe distance from it, and back away slowly. Give the snake a wide berth, and go around it. In the event that it bites you, try to remain calm and keep still. An elevated heart rate or movement will cause the venom to spread faster. Wash the wound with soapy water, and apply firm pressure to it, then seek medical attention immediately.

SUMMARY

- Prevent heat exhaustion by drinking plenty of fluids and taking precautions against the sun.
- Act swiftly to prevent heat exhaustion from escalating to heat stroke.
- Always check the weather forecast before venturing out on your hike, and pack accordingly.
- Create an action plan in case a storm suddenly comes up. This will save valuable time you could be using to get to safety.
- Do not hike during thunderstorms. Take shelter on lower ground, avoid tall trees, and remain crouched

with your feet together to prevent an indirect lightning strike from reaching you.

- Take appropriate measures to repel or avoid mosquitoes on your hike.
- While hiking at night, always take a headlamp or flashlight along, even if you don't use it to light your way. Also, take the usual safety and emergency gear with you just in case.
- Research the wildlife you may encounter on a hike, and familiarize yourself with the protocol for handling close encounters with potentially dangerous animals.

As you venture out on a hiking trip, arming yourself with knowledge about weather conditions and wildlife encounters becomes vital. From preparing for rain showers to understanding the local fauna, being well-informed enhances your hiking experience and minimizes risks. Now, let's delve into the crucial topic of hiking safely, especially when heading out on your own.

7

HIKING SAFELY

Safety is not about fear. It's about being prepared and responsible.

— UNKNOWN

SOLO HIKING SAFETY

Going out on your own for a solo hiking experience can be liberating and thrilling. However, it is crucial to prioritize safety when venturing out alone. Here are a few essential safety precautions to follow to ensure your safety when hiking solo:

- While the hiking community is overwhelmingly friendly and the likelihood of running into unsavory characters is small, it's still a good idea to be vigilant, especially if you are a woman alone.
- Take protection. In the event of a threatening wildlife encounter, have bear spray at hand. A quality knife can be handy for more than just use around the campsite. Read up on the legal restrictions of the area you are visiting, as well as when traveling by airplane.
- Prioritize your safety by letting someone know your whereabouts. Provide them with detailed information about your intended route, including the trailhead and any alternative routes you may consider. Share your expected return time as well. This way, if you do not return as scheduled, someone will be aware of your situation and can initiate appropriate action, such as contacting authorities or search and rescue teams if necessary. As an extra precaution, you can also leave these details in your vehicle for authorities to find should it become necessary to locate you. However, don't let it be visible through the window for everyone to see.
- Before setting out, research the trail thoroughly and familiarize yourself with the area. Study trail maps, read trip reports, and gather information about the terrain, potential hazards, and any required permits or regulations. Understand the trail difficulty,

elevation gain, and estimated time to complete the hike.

- When solo hiking, packing the 10 Essentials is crucial for self-sufficiency and preparedness:

1) a detailed map and compass or GPS device

2) sun protection such as sunscreen, a hat, and sunglasses

3) clothing suited to any conditions you may encounter on the hike based on the season, weather, altitude, and temperature

4) a reliable flashlight or headlamp

5) a well-stocked first-aid kit

6) a knife

7) fire starters

8) emergency shelter

9) food

10) water

(Pack extra food and water to sustain yourself in case of unexpected delays)

- Dressing appropriately for the weather and wearing sturdy, comfortable hiking shoes are important. Check the weather forecast, and choose clothing layers that provide insulation and protection from the elements. Opt for moisture-wicking fabrics to keep you dry and comfortable. Wear sturdy hiking shoes or boots that offer good traction and ankle support. This ensures stability and reduces the risk of slips, sprains, or other injuries while hiking alone.

- Ensure your phone has a full battery before setting out, and take a portable charger along to extend its lifespan. In case of emergencies, a phone can be used to call for help or communicate your location provided it has a signal. It also allows you to access navigation apps or emergency services when necessary.

- Stay on marked trails, and adhere to safety signs and guidelines. Straying from designated paths increases the risk of getting lost or encountering hazardous terrain. Follow trail markers, signposts, and any specific instructions provided. Respect any closures or restrictions in place for your safety and the preservation of the environment.

- Pace yourself, and take regular breaks to avoid exhaustion or overexertion. Listen to your body, and adjust your pace when necessary. Allow yourself time to rest and recharge, especially during long or challenging hikes. Take advantage of scenic spots or designated rest areas to hydrate, refuel, and enjoy the surroundings. Pacing and taking breaks help prevent fatigue and reduce the risk of injury.

- Don't wear headphones while hiking. Be aware of your surroundings, and take note of wildlife activity and any unusual sounds. Stay alert, and listen for signs of wildlife, such as rustling leaves or calls. This awareness helps you avoid surprising or startling animals, reducing the risk of negative encounters. Pay attention to your surroundings, including changes in the landscape or weather conditions. Being observant enhances your safety and allows you to fully appreciate the natural environment.

- Trust your instincts. If a situation feels risky or unfamiliar, it's best to err on the side of caution and avoid it, turn back, or seek an alternative route. Your safety must always take priority. Stick to well-known trails, and avoid venturing into unfamiliar, potentially dangerous areas.

- Staying hydrated is of the utmost importance when hiking solo. Drink water regularly to prevent dehydration, especially in warm or strenuous conditions. Carry an adequate supply of water, and have a plan to refill if necessary. Take small sips frequently rather than waiting until you feel thirsty. Remember that dehydration can impair judgment and physical performance. With no one else around to notice and prompt you to drink water when you're dehydrated, forming the habit of taking regular, small sips is vital.

- Carry a whistle or other signaling device as a safety precaution to increase your chances of being located quickly in the event of an emergency.

- Avoid hiking during severe weather conditions or when visibility is poor. Inclement weather can pose significant risks, such as lightning strikes, flash floods, mudslides, or avalanches. Reduced visibility increases the chances of getting disoriented or losing your way. Stay updated on weather forecasts and trail conditions before heading out. If the weather deteriorates or visibility is compromised, it is best to postpone your hike.

- Stay alert, and continuously monitor changes in weather conditions, trail conditions, and unexpected events. Keep an eye on the sky for dark clouds or sudden weather shifts. Be aware of potential hazards such as fallen trees or rock slides. Carry the necessary gear and supplies to enable you to adapt to changing circumstances. By staying alert and prepared, you can proactively respond to any challenges or unforeseen situations that may arise on your hike.

- Be cautious of wildlife encounters, and know how to react if you come across animals. Don't feed any wild animals, and always keep your distance. Familiarize yourself with the wildlife in the area, and understand their behaviors. If you encounter wildlife, remain calm, and back away slowly. Avoid sudden movements or loud noises that may provoke them. By being cautious and knowledgeable, you can peacefully coexist with wildlife and neutralize any potential threats.

- Practice Leave No Trace principles to minimize your impact on the environment and preserve the ecosystem. Carry all your trash and waste out, leaving no trace of your presence. Stay on designated trails to avoid damaging vegetation or disrupting wildlife habitats.

WHEN THE UNEXPECTED HAPPENS

Panic can easily set in when the unexpected happens and you are miles away from help. The following is a list of tips in the event that you find yourself in a difficult situation in the backcountry:

- Familiarize yourself with basic wilderness survival skills, such as building a fire, constructing a shelter, and finding edible plants.
- Prepare yourself mentally for the unexpected. Stay calm, and take care of large tasks one small step at a time.
- In the event that you become lost, remember to STOP: stop, think, observe, and plan. Stay on the trail, or backtrack to your last known location.
- If weather conditions suddenly change or you encounter a storm, seek shelter immediately to

protect yourself from rain, wind, lightning, or extreme temperatures.

- If you find yourself feeling fatigued or unwell, take regular breaks and listen to your body. Overexertion can lead to accidents and injuries.
- In case of an emergency, use a whistle, signal mirror, fire, smoke signals, or brightly colored clothing to attract attention from potential rescuers.
- If something doesn't feel right or safe, trust your instincts and make cautious decisions.
- Do not rely on your cell phone for navigation, illumination, or medical assistance. Save your phone's battery life for emergencies by switching it off or switching to airplane mode. Remember that you won't always have reception. If you manage to call for help, keep your phone on to make it easier for emergency personnel to trace your call and find you.
- Stick to paths where you have solid footing, and avoid slippery slopes.
- Avoid fast-moving water, and be very careful when crossing rivers.
- If you are hiking along the coast, be especially attentive to tidal behavior. Consult a local tide table, and don't get caught by the incoming tide; but if you do, seek higher ground and call for help.
- Make use of environmentally safe and photodegradable trail-marking ribbon to find your

way back to the trail should you veer off or, if you're lost, to make it easier for emergency personnel to find you.

- Watch your step, and practice defensive hiking. Being aware of the feeling of the terrain under your feet could give you an early warning of sudden changes, like slippery spots or loose gravel that might cause a fall.
- Be aware of how your backpack influences your movement and reflexes. A heavy pack will make it more difficult to keep your balance and also make your movements more sluggish.

SUMMARY

- Always inform someone of your plans when going on a solo hike. Be as detailed as possible so that they'll be able to raise the alarm in the event that you don't return and can provide authorities with information on your whereabouts.
- Stay on the trail to prevent getting lost and make it easier for potential rescuers to find you.
- Take regular breaks to avoid overexertion.
- Stay well hydrated at all times.
- Your cell phone is not a compass, map, or flashlight.
- Enjoy the freedom to explore, but always prioritize your safety. Be self-reliant, make informed decisions, trust your instincts, and be cautious.

- Always remember to leave no trace.

Before you take on the trails on your own, make a list of three dependable people who you can trust to know your location during a hike. Always supply them with your full itinerary.

Remember, solo hiking can be a rewarding experience filled with opportunities for personal growth and a chance to make a deeper connection with the natural world, but being cautious and prepared for the unexpected will ensure your safety and well-being while exploring the great outdoors.

CONCLUSION

As we come to the end of *The Hiker's Companion,* I hope that this journey into the world of hiking has left you with newfound confidence, knowledge, and excitement to embrace the beauty and challenges of the natural world. Congratulations, you are now equipped with the essential tools and wisdom to embark on your adventures with a spirit of adventure and preparedness.

Throughout this book, we have traversed the landscapes of preparation, safety, navigation, gear selection, and wilderness ethics. We have unveiled the secrets of selecting the right gear and extras for your expeditions, from sturdy hiking boots to trekking poles, and from emergency blankets to nutrition-packed snacks. We have delved into the art of reading topographical maps, navigating with a compass, and understanding the significance of a well-stocked first-aid kit to confidently blaze your trail.

In *The Hiker's Companion*, we have emphasized the paramount importance of safety in the great outdoors. We have illuminated the strategies to mitigate risks, from weather challenges to wildlife encounters, empowering you to make wise decisions on the trail. We have explored the art of responsible camping and the significance of Leave No Trace principles, ensuring that your footprints on the earth are gentle and respectful.

We hope you have discovered the deep connection between hiking and self-discovery. The act of wandering in the wild allows us to untether from the stresses of modern life and find solace in the embrace of nature's soothing rhythms. As you embark on your treks, you will discover that the trails offer not only a window into the splendor of the natural world but also a mirror reflecting the depths of your own soul. The challenges faced on the trail often parallel the obstacles you face in life, teaching you resilience, perseverance, and the power of mindfulness.

Remember that every step taken on the trail is a sacred journey, and the mountains and forests are not merely destinations but also sanctuaries that nurture our spirits. Embrace the serenity of nature, and cherish the moments of silence and contemplation it offers. Open your heart to the awe-inspiring beauty of sunrises over mountain peaks and sunsets painting the sky in hues of gold and crimson.

As a beginner in the great outdoors, you may face uncertainties and doubts, but always remember that every seasoned hiker was once a novice. Embrace the learning process, and let each expedition serve as a stepping stone on the path of growth and adventure. Nature is a masterful teacher, and the trails are classrooms of discovery and enlightenment. The mountains, forests, and deserts have stories to tell, and you have become a part of this timeless narrative.

In the spirit of exploration and camaraderie, I encourage you to venture into new territories, discover hidden gems, and forge connections with fellow hikers who share the same passion for nature's marvels. The hiking community is a vast and welcoming group of like-minded folks, bound together by the love of the trails and the wonders they behold.

With a blend of preparation, perseverance, and a touch of wanderlust, your path is now illuminated by the sun and stars (and the occasional headlamp), leading you to vistas unexplored and dreams yet to be realized. May your adventures be filled with joy, awe, and a deeper connection with the magnificent world around you.

So, seize your backpack, lace up your boots, and let the trails guide you onward. Your journey as a hiker has just begun, and with each step, you embark on an odyssey that will etch lasting memories into your heart, for the great outdoors is a boundless canvas on which you can paint your story of exploration and wonder.

I hope you enjoyed reading *The Hiker's Companion*. I'd love to hear your thoughts! Please consider sharing your review and feedback. Your input will continue to inspire more hikers on their wilderness journeys. Here is a link: https://www.amazon.com/review/create-review/?asin=[ASIN

Or, Visit Amazon, find The Hiker's Companion for Beginners by Quinn Marshal, click on "Write a review", share your thoughts and anything you gained from the book, and hit the"Submit" button. Thank you!

Happy hiking, and may the beauty of nature embrace you forever!

REFERENCES

AllTrails: Trail guides & maps for hiking, camping, and running. (2023). AllTrails.com. https://www.alltrails.com/

Arches National Park (U.S. National Park Service). (2016a). Nps.gov. https://www.nps.gov/arch/index.htm

Are trekking poles worth it? Pros and cons. (2022, October 26). Wheretheroadforks.com. https://wheretheroadforks.com/do-i-need-trekking-poles-pros-and-cons/

Backpacking gear list: What to bring on a backpacking trip. (2019a, February 5). Rei.com. https://www.rei.com/learn/expert-advice/backpacking-checklist.html

Backpacking in bear country. (2022, August 18). Rei.com. https://www.rei.com/learn/expert-advice/backpacking-in-bear-country.html

Bear identification. (2017). Nps.gov. https://www.nps.gov/articles/bear-identification.htm

Benefits of hiking - trails & hiking (U.S. National Park Service). (2018b, May 29). Nps.gov. https://www.nps.gov/subjects/trails/benefits-of-hiking.htm

Best lightweight backpacking food 2020. (2020). CleverHiker. https://www.cleverhiker.com/lightweight-backpacking-food-guide-meal-planning-nutrition

Best time to visit Rocky Mountain National Park. (2023). Wildland Trekking. https://wildlandtrekking.com/rocky-mountain-visitor-guide/best-time-to-visit-rocky-mountain/

Blaz. (2014, November 11). *How to plan a hiking trip?* Best Hiking. https://besthiking.net/plan-hiking-tour/

Bliss, A. (2022, July 21). *Hiking essentials checklist (26 things to pack on a hike) - Travel Lemming.* Travellemming.com. https://travellemming.com/hiking-essentials-packing-list/

Bor, K. (2020a, April 1). *Hiking alone: Solo hiking benefits and safety tips.* Bearfoot Theory. https://bearfoottheory.com/hiking-alone/

Bor, K. (2020b, May 4). *What to wear hiking: Women's guide to outdoor apparel.* Bearfoot Theory. https://bearfoottheory.com/what-to-wear-hiking/

Bor, K. (2020c, August 24). *11 benefits of hiking for health and well-being.* Bearfoot Theory. https://bearfoottheory.com/benefits-of-hiking/

Bor, K. (2021, May 10). *Best hiking a pps for finding local trails & navigation.* Bearfoot Theory. https://bearfoottheory.com/best-trail-finder-apps-websites/

Bor, K. (2023, April 13). *6 best Arches National Park hikes + tips for visiting.* Bearfoot Theory. https://bearfoottheory.com/hikes-in-arches-national-park/

Cage, C. (2017, June 24). *THE Naked Hiking Day Guide | 15 Best Photos from the Trail.* Greenbelly Meals. https://www.greenbelly.co/pages/naked-hiking

Canyonlands National Park. (2023). National Park Foundation. https://www.nationalparks.org/explore/parks/canyonlands-national-park

Capitol Reef National Park (U.S. National Park Service). (2016b). Nps.gov. https://www.nps.gov/care/index.htm

Collins, D. (2018, June 8). *Mosquitos & hiking: How to protect yourself.* Clever-Hiker. https://www.cleverhiker.com/blog/mosquitos-hiking-how-to-protect-yourself

Collins, D. (2019, November 11). *How to stay clean while backpacking.* Clever-Hiker. https://www.cleverhiker.com/blog/how-to-stay-clean-while-backpacking

Don't let these hiking scenarios derail your adventure: How to deal with the unexpected. (2022, February 2). Natural Land Institute. https://www.naturalland.org/dont-let-these-hiking-scenarios-derail-your-adventure-how-to-deal-with-the-unexpected/

Dundas, S. (2021, April 27). *Planning a hiking trip: The complete guide.* TripSavvy. https://www.tripsavvy.com/planning-a-hiking-trip-the-complete-guide-5180849

87 backpacking food ideas. (2021, March 11). Fresh off the Grid. https://www.freshoffthegrid.com/backpacking-food-ideas/

Eldridge, H. (2023, April 3). *Ultimate day hiking checklist.* CleverHiker. https://www.cleverhiker.com/blog/day-hike-checklist

Eyton, T. (2019, October 11). *16 things to do before a hike.* Happiest Outdoors. https://happiestoutdoors.ca/16-things-to-do-before-a-hike/

Eyton, T. (2020, July 16). *How to go to the bathroom on a hike | Vancouver trails.* Vancouver Trails. https://www.vancouvertrails.com/blog/bathroom-on-a-hike/

The 15 best places to go hiking - Wildland trekking blog. (2021, May 16). Wildland

Trekking. https://wildlandtrekking.com/blog/15-best-places-to-hike/

59+ hiking statistics: How many people hike In the US? (2023). (2020, November 4). Jersey Island Holidays. https://www.jerseyislandholidays.com/59-hiking-statistics/

First-aid checklist | REI expert advice. (2003). Rei.com. https://www.rei.com/learn/expert-advice/first-aid-checklist.html

Fitness tests for hikers. (2020, April 12). Summit Strength. https://www.summitstrength.com.au/blog/tft61-fitness-tests-for-hikers

Floro, K. (2019, April 3). *How to prevent and treat 7 common thru-hiking foot problems*. The Trek. https://thetrek.co/prevent-treat-7-common-thru-hiking-foot-problems

Garay, E. (2023). *What to Wear Hiking*. Www.rei.com. https://www.rei.com/learn/expert-advice/how-to-choose-hiking-clothes.html

Gates, Z. (2023, May 19). *What to wear for your first dayhike*. Backpacker. https://www.backpacker.com/skills/what-to-wear-hiking/

Goldbach, J. (2006, April 28). *How to use a compass*. WikiHow; wikiHow. https://www.wikihow.com/Use-a-Compass

Goldhorn, C. (2017, April 20). *Put a knot around your finger: Easily forgotten backpacking gear*. The Trek. https://thetrek.co/put-knot-around-finger-easily-forgotten-backpacking-gear/

Gore, W. L. & Associates. (2017). *How to build the best hiking first aid kit*. Gore-Tex.com. https://www.gore-tex.com/blog/hiking-first-aid-kit

Gore, W. L. & Associates. (2023). *What to do if you get lost hiking | GORE-TEX brand*. Gore-Tex.com. https://www.gore-tex.com/blog/what-to-do-if-you-get-lost-hiking

Gray wolf safety. (2023). Western Wildlife Outreach. https://westernwildlife.org/gray-wolf-canis-lupus/wolf-saftey/

Hall, S. (2020, April 22). *Is it dangerous to hike at night? (13 safety tips)*. Trailand-Summit. https://trailandsummit.com/is-it-dangerous-to-hike-at-night/

Hazzard, C. (2016, December 2). *Do I need trekking poles?* HikingGuy.com. https://hikingguy.com/how-to-hike/do-i-need-trekking-poles/

Hike smart (U.S. National Park Service). (2018a). Nps.gov. https://www.nps.gov/articles/hiking-safety.htm

Hiking - Great Smoky Mountains National Park (U.S. National Park Service). (2023a). Nps.gov. https://www.nps.gov/grsm/planyourvisit/hiking.htm

Hiking: What to do in case of a storm? | La Balaguère. (2023). Purelypyrenees.com.

https://www.purelypyrenees.com/le-mag/advice/hiking-what-do-case-storm.html

Hiking checklist: What to bring on a hike. (2019b, July 31). Rei.com. https://www.rei.com/learn/expert-advice/day-hiking-checklist.html

Hiking in Capitol Reef National Park. (2023). Primary-Utahddm.simpleviewcms.com. https://primary-utahddm.simpleviewcms.com/destinations/national-parks/capitol-reef-national-park/things-to-do/hiking

Hiking 101 - the essential hiking gear list. (2023). She Dreams of Alpine. https://www.shedreamsofalpine.com/blog/2018/1/11/hiking-101-the-essential-hiking-gear-list

Hiking tips and tricks | How to plan and prepare for a hike | KOA Camping blog. (2023, May 8). Koa.com. https://koa.com/blog/hiking-tips-and-tricks-how-to-plan-and-prepare-for-a-hike/

Hot weather hiking. (2013c, April 11). American Hiking Society. https://americanhiking.org/resources/hot-weather-hiking/

How to avoid getting eaten alive by mosquitoes and ticks for hikers – outdoor adventure travel guides & tips . (2020, June 20). Thisbigwildworld.com. https://www.thisbigwildworld.com/avoid-mosquitoes-and-ticks-for-hikers/

How to read a topographic map for hiking | Backroads. (2023). Backroads.com. https://www.backroads.com/pro-tips/hiking/how-to-read-a-topographic-map-for-hiking

How to use a compass. (2013a, April 10). American Hiking Society. https://americanhiking.org/resources/how-to-use-a-compass/

Hudetz, N. (2023, May 30). *How to take care of your feet when hiking and backpacking.* Treeline Review. https://www.treelinereview.com/learn-skills/foot-care-hiking-backpacking

If you get lost | US Forest Service. (2020). Usda.gov. https://www.fs.usda.gov/visit/know-before-you-go/if-you-get-lost

Inspiring quotes about nature. (2023, June 19). Southern Living Editors. *Southern Living.* https://www.southernliving.com/culture/nature-quotes

Jones, J. (2021, January 10). *This is the absolute best time to visit Zion National Park.* Well Planned Journey. https://www.wellplannedjourney.com/best-time-to-visit-zion-national-park/

Joshua Tree National Park (U.S. National Park Service). (2023b). Nps.gov. https://www.nps.gov/jotr/index.htm

Kachroo-Levine, M. (2021, June 17). *The best hikes in every state.* Travel +

Leisure. https://www.travelandleisure.com/trip-ideas/nature-travel/where-to-go-hiking-near-me

Kilpatrick, T. (2023, July 6). *From reducing strain to helping casualties, there's no end to the reasons to carry hiking poles.* The Manual. https://www.themanual.com/outdoors/do-i-need-trekking-poles/

Kim, D. (2019, June 27). *What to do if you get lost hiking.* Sunset Magazine. https://www.sunset.com/travel/outdoor-adventure/how-to-survive-if-you-get-lost-hiking

Larson, T. (2023). *Wildlife safety tips.* Rei.com. https://www.rei.com/learn/expert-advice/wildlife-safety-tips.html

Leong, J. (2022, June 21). *How to read a map: Find your way in the great outdoors.* Advnture.com. https://www.advnture.com/how-to/how-to-read-a-map

Lightning safety. (2013d, April 11). American Hiking Society. https://americanhiking.org/resources/lightning-safety

McIntosh-Tolle, L. (2019, July 8). *How to use a compass: Compass/map navigation.* Rei.com. https://www.rei.com/learn/expert-advice/navigation-basics.html

Meal planning for backpacking. (2023). Rei.com. https://www.rei.com/learn/expert-advice/planning-menu.html

Mixell, A. (2021, March 25). *11 tips for safely hiking alone as a woman.* Explorer Chick. https://explorerchick.com/journal/women-safely-hiking-alone-tips/

Morgan, M. & Morgan, K. (2021, November 23). *23 best hikes In Mt Rainier National Park for 2023.* Where Are Those Morgans. https://wherearethosemorgans.com/best-hikes-in-mt-rainier-national-park/

Morgan, M., & Morgan, K. (2020, June 18). *Yellowstone itinerary 4 days: The ultimate first time visitor guide.* Where Are Those Morgans. https://wherearethosemorgans.com/yellowstone-itinerary-4-days/

Morgan, M., & Morgan, K. (2022a, January 17). *Best time to visit Grand Canyon National Park by month and season.* Where Are Those Morgans. https://wherearethosemorgans.com/best-time-to-visit-grand-canyon-national-park/

Morgan, M., & Morgan, K. (2022b, March 9). *20 best hikes In Zion National Park for 2023.* Where Are Those Morgans. https://wherearethosemorgans.com/best-hikes-in-zion-national-park/

Mueller, S. (2020, February 1). *60 awesome baseball quotes. Planet of Success.*

https://www.planetofsuccess.com/blog/2017/baseball-quotes/

Nature - Zion National Park (U.S. National Park Service). (2023c). Nps.gov. https://www.nps.gov/zion/learn/nature/index.htm

9 benefits of hiking. (2022, November 30). Cleveland Clinic. https://health.cleve landclinic.org/9-benefits-of-hiking/

Olson, K. (2022, August 23). *Why do people like hiking? [15 great reasons]*. The Hiking Helper. https://thehikinghelper.com/why-do-people-like-hiking/

Panaro, J. (2020, September 17). *13 tips | how to find hiking trails wherever you are [2021]*. Honestly Modern. https://www.honestlymodern.com/how-to-find-hiking-trails/

Pattiz, A. (2022, November 14). *6 breathtaking hikes in Bryce Canyon National Park*. Embrace Someplace. https://embracesomeplace.com/bryce-canyon-best-hikes/

Planning your hike. (2013b, April 10). American Hiking Society. https://ameri canhiking.org/resources/planning-your-hike/

Plot your loop: Tips for researching your own routes. (2023). Washington Trails Association. https://www.wta.org/go-outside/new-to-hiking/plot-your-loop-tips-for-researching-your-own-routes

Quotes about hiking: 120+ best hiking quotes to inspire you · we dream of travel blog. (2020, September 28). We Dream of Travel Blog. https://www.wedreamof travel.com/quotes-about-hiking/

Recognizing and preventing heat stroke when hiking. (2018, July 25). Bryce Canyon. https://www.brycecanyon.net/recognizing-and-preventing-heat-stroke-when-hiking/

Rowan. (2021, January 28). *A simple hiking fitness test*. Summit Strength. https://www.summitstrength.com.au/blog/a-simple-hiking-fitness-test

Roy, A. (2023, June 7). *How to salvage your hiking trip when you've forgotten gear*. Backpacker. https://www.backpacker.com/skills/beginner-skills/pack ing/salvage-trip-missing-hiking-gear

S., R. (2021, December 9). *A history of hiking: The driving force behind our footprints*. Silverlight. https://silverlight.store/history-of-hiking/

Sein, L. (2020, July 7). *What to do if you are caught in a thunderstorm while hiking*. Cortazu. https://cortazu.com/blogs/news/what-to-do-if-you-are-caught-in-a-thunderstorm-while-hiking

Shelly. (2023, May 24). *The best time to visit Death Valley*. Almost There Adventures. https://almostthereadventures.com/best-time-to-visit-death-valley/

Snapper, E. (2016, June 27). *Charitable MLB players. Fanatics Forum.* https://blog.fanatics.com/giving-back-mlb/

Spicer, D. (2023). *Solo hiking tips: How to stay safe on any trail as a female hiker.* Hiking for Her. https://www.hiking-for-her.com/solo-hiking-tips.html

Steele, L. (2017, December 4). *Happy nude hiking day! Here's how to (legally) make the most of it.* Men's Journal. https://www.mensjournal.com/adventure/happy-nude-hiking-day-heres-how-to-legally-make-the-most-of-it-w489096

A storm in the mountains, what should you do? (2023). Quechua.com. https://www.quechua.com/a-storm-in-the-mountains-what-should-you-do

Thomas, L. (2023). *A pro hiker shares 6 best hikes in Yosemite National Park.* 57hours - Discover Amazing Outdoor Adventures. https://57hours.com/best-of/yosemite-hikes/

Tips for hiking in the heat and preventing heatstroke. (2023). Limitlesshiker. https://www.limitlesshiker.com/blog/tips-for-hiking-in-the-heat-and-preventing-heatstroke/

Trekking poles & hiking staffs: How to choose. (2018, May 11). Rei.com. https://www.rei.com/learn/expert-advice/trekking-poles-hiking-staffs.html

Vukovic, D. (2022, May 6). *Backpacking? 12 things you forgot to pack (or didn't pack on purpose but should have!).* Mom Goes Camping. https://momgoescamping.com/backpacking-gear-forgot-pack/

Welton, L. (2022, January 21). *This fitness test can tell you how strong of a hiker you are—and how to get fitter.* Backpacker. https://www.backpacker.com/skills/backpacking-fitness/this-step-test-helps-hikers-train-better/

Werner, P. (2022, November 7). *How to stay clean on a backpacking trip.* SectionHiker.com. https://sectionhiker.com/how-to-stay-clean-backpacking/

What are the different types of hiking? 16 you should know. (2022, September 29). Kenver. https://kenver.com/blogs/news/16-hiking-types

What is hiking? (2023). Rookieroad.com. https://www.rookieroad.com/hiking/what-is/

What is the best season to visit? - Death Valley National Park (U.S. National Park Service). (2016c). Nps.gov. https://www.nps.gov/deva/planyourvisit/seasons.htm

What to do if you get lost hiking | Mountain safety |Expert advice. (2021, September 24). Inside the Outdoors | Mountain Warehouse Community. https://www.mountainwarehouse.com/expert-advice/what-to-do-if-you-get-lost-hiking

Why do people actually go hiking? 4 reasons that sum it up. (2008, October 17). Thrillspire. https://thrillspire.com/why-do-people-go-hiking

Yuko, E. (2020, July 11). *How to read a trail map.* Lifehacker. https://lifehacker.com/how-to-read-a-trail-map-1844344804

www.ingramcontent.com/pod-product-compliance
Lightning Source LLC
Chambersburg PA
CBHW022054020426
42335CB00012B/691